ASSESSING LANGUAGE PRODUCTION IN CHILDREN

ASSESSING LANGUAGE PRODUCTION IN CHILDREN: EXPERIMENTAL PROCEDURES, by Jon F. Miller, Ph.D., is the inaugural volume of the **Assessing Communicative Behavior Series**—Jon F. Miller, Ph.D., series editor.

Published volumes:

PROCEDURES FOR THE PHONOLOGICAL ANALYSIS OF CHILDREN'S LANGUAGE
David Ingram, Ph.D.

Volumes in preparation:

ASSESSING LANGUAGE COMPREHENSION IN CHILDREN: Experimental Procedures
Jon F. Miller, Ph.D.

ASSESSING COGNITIVE PERFORMANCE: Piagetian Procedures
Roberta Dihoff, Ph.D.

ASSESSING COMMUNICATIVE PERFORMANCE: Pragmatic Considerations

Assessing Language Production in Children: Experimental Procedures is the third revision of a manual of informal language assessment procedures developed at the Waisman Center on Mental Retardation and Human Development.

Deep acknowledgment is extended to the people listed on the opposite page for their kind permission to reproduce their procedures in this volume.

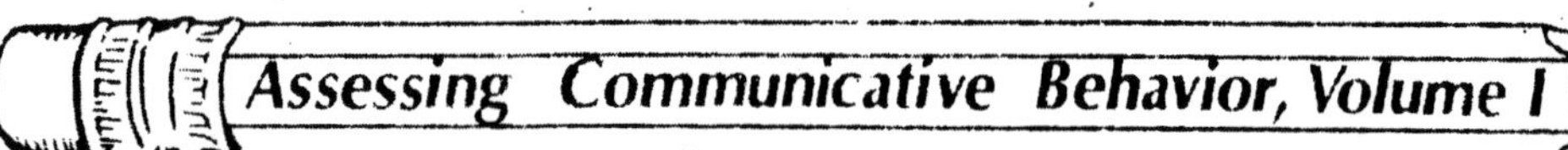

ASSESSING LANGUAGE PRODUCTION IN CHILDREN

EXPERIMENTAL PROCEDURES

Jon F. Miller, Ph.D.

Professor and Section Head
Communicative Disorders
Waisman Center on Mental Retardation
and Human Development

with chapters by

Thomas M. Klee, M.A. and **Rhea Paul, M.A.**
Department of Communicative Disorders

and

Robin S. Chapman, Ph.D.
Professor of Communicative Disorders
University of Wisconsin-Madison

and contributions and procedures by

Ursula Bellugi
Robin S. Chapman
Carol Goossens
Ellen Green
Susan Marks
Helene Frye-Osier
Rhea Paul
Joe Reichle
Susan Schmidt
Shelley Schwimmer Gluck
Shelly Werner
David E. Yoder

ALLYN AND BACON
Boston London Sydney Toronto Tokyo Singapore

A Pearson Education Company
160 Gould Street
Needham Heights, Massachusetts 02194

ISBN 0-205-13546-3

Printed in the United States of America

10 9 8 7 95 94 93 92 91

Contents

Preface

In this volume, we have gathered together a variety of experimental procedures to be used by clinicians for assessing productive language behavior in children. The procedures come from our clinical experience in applying the research literature to the task of assessing developmentally disabled children at the Waisman Center on Mental Retardation and Human Development, University of Wisconsin–Madison.

Over the past six years we have directed our efforts to discovering techniques and strategies that clarified the communicative characteristics and problems of our population of developmentally disabled children. The children have taught us that assessment protocols must be individualized for each child, that multiple means to assess the same behavior are necessary, and that experimental nonstandardized, informal, criterion-referenced procedures are frequently our best source of information. This volume presents the procedures we have found useful in evaluating productive language performance.

Our major goal is the developmental description of productive language. In our clinical experience, most children with language problems can be best described as "delayed." However, deviant language, like delayed language, cannot be identified unless it is examined carefully through a developmental model. Therefore, effective use of the procedures presented here is dependent upon the reader's familiarity with and understanding of the literature on normal language development. This manual itself is not an adequate source of preliminary information on normal language acquisition. Many forms of shorthand for describing developmental data have been used on the assumption that the reader has a foundational knowledge of the normal sequence of language development. Then, too, the developmental data presented for interpretive purposes will change, becoming more specific with new research. So, clinicians using the manual will find it necessary to augment the information presented here with data from the most recent research literature.

This volume is intended as a reference for procedures, content selection, and interpretation criteria necessary for the informal evaluation of language behavior. It is important that procedures and content be adapted to each child individually. In this respect, the procedures discussed should be used as guidelines rather than measures applicable to all children. For specific expectations and procedures applicable to a particular population—such as an unusually high socioeconomic group or a Hispanic population—normative data for that group should be collected. We have attempted to provide here a model of informal assessment that could be used with reference to any set of normative expectations.

This volume is the first in a series devoted to the compilation of experimental clinical assessment procedures. The second volume assembles procedures to evaluate phonological performance in children and the third to evaluate children's language comprehension. Subsequent volumes explore assessment procedures for evaluating cognitive performance from a Piagetian perspective, and the use of language for communicative purposes. Each volume presents a multidimensional approach to assessment and includes a variety of procedures to describe performance status. This multidimensional approach is directed toward describing developmentally significant achievements. Each volume provides the means to determine if a problem exists, the nature and scope of the problem, as well as the explicit description of performance necessary to determine the mode and content of intervention. The first five volumes will provide the means for describing multiple performance deficits both within and among production, comprehension, and pragmatic processes as they relate to cognitive status.

The volumes of this series are the descendants of two previous working drafts produced at the Waisman Center. The first of these drafts, produced in 1974, was entitled *A Developmental Approach Toward Assessing Communication Behavior in Children: A Reference Manual of Ongoing Theoretical and Methodological Advancements.* The second draft, completed in 1976, was entitled *Procedures for Assessing Children's Language: A Developmental Process Approach.* As the title got shorter the volume got longer. Both of these volumes, originally constructed for student training, proved quite useful as clinical reference manuals. With the rapid expansion of the state of the art, our procedures have expanded and now require a series of volumes, each devoted to a single process or goal.

A number of individuals have made significant contributions to this volume and I would like to take this opportunity to express my thanks and appreciation to them. For the past six years, Robin Chapman and Dave Yoder have given freely of their time and ideas, reading and making substantive comments on previous drafts and providing continuing support for this project. The students in my seminar over the past three years have provided not only the incentive to complete this volume but also numerous ideas and procedures, many of which can be found in the text. I would particularly like to thank Truman Coggins, Gary Gill, Peggy Rosin, Nat Owings, Margaret McMillen, Deb Eng, Rhea Paul, Tom Klee, Chris Dollaghan, Joe Reichle, Jean Thomson, and Larry Kohn for their substantive comments and contributions to this work. In addition, I am indebted to Judith Johnston, Peter Hixon, and Laurence Leonard, who provided substantive and detailed reviews of an early draft of this volume. Their insights, for which I am very grateful, added significantly to the clarity and organization.

Finally, I would like to thank the children and their families who, in coming to the Waisman Center, have taught us so much.

ASSESSING LANGUAGE PRODUCTION IN CHILDREN

INTRODUCTION

Assessing Difficult-to-Test Children

Contents

With the implementation of PL 94-142, multidisciplinary teams are faced with the task of evaluating, summarizing, and interpreting data on children from a number of sources. Individualized education programs (IEPs) must be written incorporating developmental status data with learning and performance descriptions. It is clear that the psychologist, the speech-language pathologist, the teacher, and other professionals must coordinate their efforts to develop appropriate IEPs. The assessment procedures and descriptive format to be presented in this Assessing Communicative Behavior Series should prove a useful tool in this cooperative effort to meet the communication needs of the developmentally disabled child.

The purpose of the format of describing language behavior presented in this volume is to identify language delay or disorder in children with a variety of handicapping conditions. In order to do this, an approach to assessment developed for multiply handicapped, developmentally disabled children is discussed. Both what to assess and how to assess it are considered. Particular emphasis is placed on the necessity of having nonverbal measures of cognitive development for interpreting the language behavior of this population. The resulting descriptive format provides a summary mechanism for quantifying language delay or disorders, as well as a means of describing language behavior across children, or within the same child, over time.

A DEVELOPMENTAL PHILOSOPHY OF ASSESSMENT

The first step in describing language behavior is to find an approach to assessment for the population under study that quantifies valid indices of performance. The problems of assessing, describing, and interpreting language performance are particularly difficult in developmentally disabled children because of their wide ranges of performance. Frequently, the children are profoundly retarded and have multiply handicapping conditions. The approach to the assessment of these children that evolved at the Waisman Center on Mental Retardation and Human Development, University of Wisconsin-Madison is fundamentally developmental. It focuses on defining and describing the developmental status of the child for each of the basic language processes (Miller, 1978). Assessment procedures are individualized for each child, but always evaluate linguistic achievements within the basic processes of comprehension, production, and use of language for communication. The major premise of this approach is that no child is untestable; all children behave in some regular or usual fashion. This is a positive approach to assessment, directed toward describing what the child *can* do, resulting in as complete a description as possible from which interpretive judgments can be made. We believe that decisions regarding the presence or absence of a language delay or disorder cannot be made in this population without a complete description of the developmental status of the child's comprehension, production, and use of language for communication. The role of cognitive development in making these decisions is the subject of the latter half of this introduction.

What to Assess

Given the complex nature of language and communicative behavior, there are a number of structural and functional aspects of the system to be assessed. The linguistic dimensions of our behavioral description are found in Table 1. The validity of these behaviors for our descriptive format is derived from two sources. First, each represents a distinct, measurable component of the linguistic system, observable in comprehension, production, or discourse (Miller, 1978). Second, children designated as language disordered demonstrate deficit performance in one or more of these aspects of the language system (Miller, Chapman, and Bedrosian, 1977; Bloom and Lahey, 1978; Leonard, 1978).

The aspects selected for assessment are essential to the communicative use of the language system. However, it should be pointed out that these categories represent only those for which acquisition has been documented. Descriptions of the child's advancing communicative abilities are far from complete. The more that researchers learn about language acquisition, the older becomes the child identified as having adult competence, particularly conversational competence (Bowerman, 1978). As further developmental and experimental research is done, components will need to be added to the descriptive format.

The processes and linguistic elements listed in Table 1 represent a minimal set of data points needed to document a child's developmental status. The intent of this documentation is to provide a precise description of developmental status. Obviously, this is only part of a complete view of a child's performance. It ignores processing strategies, learning styles, and initiating and responding characteristics in interactions. However, it is the logical starting point. Without status data, descriptions of processing and learning strategies would be difficult to interpret. Clearly these performance and learning characteristics are important, but only as they relate to the child's developmental status, by pointing the way to possible explanations for current status and potentially facilitative approaches to intervention.

Table 1. Processes assessed as the bases for describing language performance

1. ***Comprehension*** Understanding of linguistic units
   A. *Vocabulary* Word meanings
   B. *Syntax—semantics* Grammatical structure and meaning not separable in assessing comprehension
2. ***Production*** Producing linguistic elements
   A. *Syntax* Sentence structure, grammatical elements
   B. *Semantics* Sentence meaning, lexical meaning
   C. *Phonology* Sound elements and rules for ordering in English
3. ***Communication*** Use of language
   A. *Communication functions and intentions*

This chapter is reprinted, with adaptations, from Jon F. Miller, 1978, Identifying language disorders in retarded children, School Psychology Digest, 7(4):27–44, by permission.

How to Assess Language

In general, we have used three different types of procedures designed to assess language behavior: 1) standardized tests or normatively based procedures evaluating one or more linguistic dimensions (see Siegel and Broen, 1976, for an informative review); 2) developmental scales—where major developmental achievements are sampled through an adult informant or through child activities; and 3) nonstandardized or informal procedures, including directed behavioral observations. These are criterion-referenced procedures using experimental developmental data from normal subjects for interpretation.

Each of these procedural types has its own particular application depending upon the child to be assessed and the behaviors to be evaluated. These procedural types are not mutually exclusive. The complete evaluation of a child will often require one or more specific procedures from each of the three types listed. The decision to use a particular procedure obviously depends on many factors, including the developmental level of the child, the information sought, and the perceptual and motor status of the child.

The specific procedures we have found most useful with our populations are listed by the linguistic process and dimension assessed.

Comprehension of Syntax This category is assessed with the Miller-Yoder Test of Grammatical Comprehension (1972); the Test for Auditory Comprehension of Language (Carrow, 1973); the Northwest Syntax Screening Test (Lee, 1971); and Answers to Questions and Responses to Commands and Locatives (Miller, 1976). Object manipulation procedures are also used. Early development is assessed in natural context with procedures similar to those of Huttenlocher (1974) and of Sachs and Truswell (1976). Interpretation is provided by data from normal children (Miller, Chapman, Branston, Reichle, 1980).

Comprehension of Vocabulary This category is assessed with the Peabody Picture Vocabulary Test and the Boehm Basic Concept Inventory. In early development, object names and verbs (familiar and unfamiliar) are assessed in context, within and outside of the child's visual field. Interpretation of the early data is provided by data from normal children (Miller, Chapman, Branston, and Reichle, 1980).

Production—Free-Speech Sample and Mean Length of Utterance (MLU)

A. A free-speech sample is recorded on audiotape or videotape. Three situations are used when possible:
   1. 15 minutes with mother in free play
   2. 15 minutes with clinician in free play
   3. 15 minutes with clinician directing child with questions and commands

B. A transcript is then written, including all speech directed to the child with contextual notes. Procedures follow those detailed in Chapter 1, this volume.

C. Mean length of utterance is computed for the first two situations using Brown's (1973) rules with a few modifications (see Chapter 2, this volume).

D. Test ages corresponding to MLU scores are derived from values predicted by a linear regression of MLU on age (n=123). Detailed discussion is found in Chapter 2, this volume.

E. The predicted values reported should be considered midpoints of ranges; e.g., ±6 months. These predicted values provide the basis for comparing production performance with comprehension, cognition, and communication.

Production—Syntax, Level of Structural Development

A. The level of structural development is determined by segmenting the transcript by construction type to note noun phrase, verb phrase, and auxiliary development; negation; and questions, both yes/no and Wh-types. (See Criteria for Assigning Structural Stage, Appendix B to Chapter 2, this volume.)

B. Charts summarizing the developmental data from research studies are organized for each construction by developmental stage (Brown, 1973). These charts serve as criteria for making stage determinations for each construction type independently.

C. Test ages for the stage determinations are derived from the MLU-age predictions. Usually age ranges are reported. Although these reflect differential development across construction types, it is not unusual to find ± one stage of development across construction types in normal children.

Production—Semantics The semantic aspects of production assessed are semantic relations (Brown, 1973) and the 14 grammatical morphemes (Brown, 1973; de Villiers and de Villiers, 1973b). As with the other production categories, the research data available on these semantic dimensions are charted to serve as criteria for interpreting individual performance (see Chapter 2, this volume).

Production—Phonology Data reported in this category are derived from a variety of articulatory proficiency measures and phonological process analyses according to Ingram (1976) and to Shriberg and Kwiatkowski (1980).

Use of Language in Communication This category is limited at the present to the assessment of communication functions or intentions, for example, requests for information, action, clarification, or attention; commenting; etc. Sets of categories for coding utterance intentions have been developed from the work of Dore (1974, 1975) and Bates (1976). Communicative development is currently the subject of a great deal of research that may soon lead to more complete descriptions of developing conversational competence. (A detailed discussion of taxonomies of communication functions is found in Chapter 4, this volume.)

THE ROLE OF COGNITIVE PERFORMANCE IN INTERPRETING LANGUAGE BEHAVIOR

With this overview of the basic content and procedures to be assessed, the framework for describing the language behavior of retarded children has been set. The linguistic elements—syntax, semantics, and phonology—need to be evaluated as they function in comprehension and production. Utterance intentions must be evaluated as an index of the use of language for communication. At this point we are left with a set of data describing the developmental status of language performance. How are we to interpret the adequacy of these behaviors? Given normal intelligence, chronological age might be used as the basis for interpreting performance. What metric is appropriate for the child with cognitive deficits?

LANGUAGE DEVELOPMENT IN THE MENTALLY RETARDED

The current view of the language performance of retarded children holds that they acquire language in the same sequence as normal children but at a slower rate (Yoder and Miller, 1972; Berry, 1976; Miller, Chapman, and Bedrosian, 1977). The implications of this view are that cognitive performance plays a role in the rate of language acquisition and that although retarded children are quite diverse in etiological classification and degree of severity, the sequence of their language development is similar to normal children. We could conclude that all retarded children exhibit delays in language acquisition relative to chronological age. This view, of course, ignores the role of cognitive development made apparent by the cognitive deficits and the correspondingly slow rate of language acquisition of retarded children.

COGNITIVE DEVELOPMENT IN THE MENTALLY RETARDED

Zigler (1969) discusses three major theoretical views of cognitive deficits in mental retardation: developmental, difference, and defect. The developmental theory of cognitive deficits postulates the differences in cognitive development between normal and retarded populations to be entirely quantitative. At any stage of development the retarded child is comparable in cognitive functioning to a chronologically younger, normal child. The empirical support for this view can be found in the studies of Woodward (1959, 1961), Inhelder (1966, 1968, 1976), Wohlhueter and Sindberg (1975), Kahn (1976), Rogers (1977), and McManis (1970). In this view the best available approximation of a given cognitive stage is a mental age score based on the measurement of a diverse set of mental abilities like the Stanford-Binet. The majority of the research findings of the language development of retarded populations is predicted by the developmental theory of cognitive deficits, i.e., same sequence, slower rate. The question remains as to how mental age as an indicator of cognitive development is related to language acquisition in retarded populations.

RELATIONS BETWEEN LANGUAGE AND COGNITIVE DEVELOPMENT IN NORMAL CHILDREN

Among normal children, a number of language milestones have been observed at similar ages or in similar sequences. Age of acquisition, invariant sequencing, and rate differences have been explained, in part, by invoking the Cognition Hypothesis. The Cognition Hypothesis argues that a particular conceptual achievement, or mental age, is necessary to a related linguistic achievement (Bloom, 1970, 1973; Brown, 1973; Cromer, 1974, 1976). Cognitive development is seen as the major pacer of the development of communication skills. Experience, linguistic input, perceptual salience, already acquired forms, and reinforcing consequences all play their roles only within the limits set by the child's cognitive status (Slobin, 1973, Chapman and Miller, 1980).

Strong Form of Cognition Hypothesis

In its strong form, the Cognition Hypothesis asserts that a given cognitive level is sufficient for the associated level of language development, except in cases of severe linguistic deprivation or significant sensory or motor deficits.

Bowerman (1974, p. 207) has listed some cognitive factors believed to be necessary for language acquisition:

1. The ability to use symbols to represent objects and events that may not be perceptually present.
2. The development of basic cognitive structures and operations.
   a. The ability to order spatially and temporally.
   b. The ability to classify in action.
   c. The ability to embed action patterns into each other.
   d. The establishment of concepts of basic invariance involving object permanence and conservation.
   e. The ability to apprehend relationships between objects and action.
   f. The construction of a model of perceptual space with certain properties.
3. The ability to derive strategies for processing linguistic material from general cognitive structures and processes that are isomorphic to aspects of language structure, and/or form the developmental sequences in which language-relevant cognitive knowledge is acquired on the linguistic level.
4. The ability to formulate appropriate concepts or categories to serve as the structural components upon which linguistic rules can operate. Neither the exact nature of these early cognitive categories nor the ways in which they change over time is yet known.

The implication of the strong form of the Cognition Hypothesis for retarded populations is that we would expect all children, with adequate linguistic experience and no perceptual or speech motor control deficits, to have developed language consistent with their mental age. If this view is correct we would not expect to find children with language development advanced relative to mental age nor would we expect to find delays relative to mental age. This view is consistent with the developmental theory of cognitive deficits.

Weak Form of Cognition Hypothesis

An alternative form of the Cognition Hypothesis, the weak form, proposes cognitive attainments as necessary but not sufficient to account for all linguistic attainment. Cromer (1976) has expressed this view:

> . . . Although the study of cognitive structures and operations and the cognitions to which they give rise are of central importance in understanding the language acquisition process, these cognitive entities by themselves are not sufficient to explain that process. Our abilities to "make available," so to speak, certain meanings to be encoded, must also possess certain specifically linguistic capabilities in order to express these meanings in language (Cromer, 1976, p. 326).

If the weak form of the Cognition Hypothesis is correct, then we would expect language development to be equal to or less than mental age in retarded populations. This view is consistent with the defect and difference theories of cognitive deficits.

Correlational Hypothesis

A third view of the relationship between cognitive and language measures, which also holds that they will be strongly associated, might be termed the Correlational Hypothesis. This hypothesis states that common maturational or cognitive factors underlie developmental sequences in both domains, but language measures are just as likely as cognitive ones to reflect change first. Brown (1973) and Bates et al. (1977) have made this more conservative proposal of relationship between the domains, Brown under the guise of attributing rate of language acquisition to a factor of general intelligence and Bates in a discussion of "local homologies," or shared features in cognitive and linguistic tasks. The Correlational Hypothesis is consistent with some, but not frequent, variation between language and cognitive levels in *either* direction.

CLINICAL IMPLICATIONS IF LANGUAGE PROBLEMS ARE DEFINED RELATIVE TO COGNITIVE LEVEL (Mental Age)

To the extent that some version of the Cognition or the Correlational Hypothesis is correct, a set of expectations for language development based on mental age performance is provided, assuming that the cognitive tasks are nonverbal. The confirmation of the metric, mental age, as the interpretive basis would allow language delay and disorders to be identified similarly in both normal and retarded populations. Language skills that are advanced, equal to, or atypical of cognitive status can be identified. These four patterns of language-cognitive relationship would lead to four quite different clinical conclusions (Miller, Chapman, and Bedrosian, 1977):

1. Cognition and language equal. Conclusion: no specific language disorder.
2. Language delayed relative to cognitive development. Conclusion: language delay exists, intensive developmental therapy is indicated.
3. Language advanced over cognitive performance. Conclusion: incorrectness of the Cognition Hypothesis for the accelerated language domain. The finding would point to the efficiency of particular language learning experiences.
4. Language atypical of cognitive skills, e.g., gross asynchrony in development of linguistic categories within a process: comprehension, production, or language use. Conclusion: language disorder exists. Child's own system needs careful, detailed evaluation.

The confirmation of some form of the Cognition or Correlational Hypothesis would provide an invaluable clinical tool, a descriptive framework through which the language performance of retarded populations can be quantified and interpreted. Types of language disorder cannot be illuminated simply by finding differences in the language performance of normal and retarded children of the same mental age.

WHERE DO WE GO FROM HERE?

The preceding overview of our approach to evaluating children's language behavior emphasizes the need for performance data across three processes: production, comprehension, and nonverbal cognitive status. While all three are integrally related, each needs to be evaluated independently, with the resultant data considered together for decision making. This first volume, detailing production assessment, only addresses one-third of the assessment problem, artificially segmenting the process into digestible units. Comprehension and cognition process will be taken up in future volumes.

This volume on language production presents assessment procedures based on behavioral observation otherwise known as informal or nonstandardized procedures. These procedures have been developed over the years, out of necessity, to baseline children's language production performance regardless of handicapping condition. These measures are not screening procedures; indeed, given our perspective, no single measure can adequately "screen" children for potential communicative handicaps. In our experience the measures presented are appropriate for documenting baseline performance and monitoring progress within language intervention programs.

Assessment remains the most difficult challenge of our field. This first volume in the series represents the beginning of a dialogue between clinicians and researchers, resulting in new models and methods for improved services to the communicatively handicapped. Please share with us your successes and failures so we may move ahead together in our quest for understanding.

SECTION I

PRODUCTIVE LANGUAGE: Free Speech

The four chapters in this section present an exploratory approach to analyzing free-speech samples, which provide quantitative data for describing productive language performance. Using these methods will result in detailed descriptions of productive language that can be compared to age expectations when developmental data are available for establishing such norms. The measures included provide for quantifying developmental status, describing structural, semantic, and pragmatic characteristics, and noting variability of performance within and between speech samples.

Each of the four chapters examines one aspect of evaluating children's spontaneous speech. Chapter 1 is an overview of clinical considerations addressing problems of sampling, interaction style, context, transcription format, and relationships among various analysis procedures. Specific analysis procedures for evaluating syntactic and semantic components of free-speech samples are detailed in Chapter 2. A case study comparing six syntactic analysis procedures is presented in Chapter 3. In Chapter 4 a detailed discussion of the development of intentional communication skills is presented. Taxonomies of communicative intent are presented and discussed relative to their defining properties and their relationship to structural and semantic characteristics of the language. The clinical exploration of intentional communication is discussed at each level of development.

CHAPTER 1

Collecting and Recording Speech Samples

Contents

The evaluation of children's productive language through free-speech sample analysis is one of the most revealing procedures available to us. First, it makes the child's stream of speech accessible. When the child's speech is in written form, we can get our hands on it and manipulate it through subsequent analysis. Second, it is revealing because we can check and confirm our judgments. We can score and categorize the same utterances on multiple quantitative and qualitative dimensions. Not only do multiple analyses of a transcript provide a degree of economy, but they also allow us to evaluate the interaction between analysis categories.

Two major processes are involved in analyzing children's free-speech samples. The first is collecting and recording a reliable speech sample. The second is the actual analysis of the child's utterances. Without careful consideration of the first process, the second will result in questionable or meaningless information about the child's productive language capacity because free-speech sample analyses are only as good as the transcripts from which they come. The transcript should reflect the way the child usually talks and what he or she talks about.

COLLECTING AND RECORDING A REPRESENTATIVE SAMPLE

Children usually talk to make requests, demands, or comments to other people about things they want or things that interest them. They respond to the requests or comments made by other people. They are not likely, however, to converse with a tape recorder, which has minimal response capabilities and little of interest to say. It is our job as clinicians to elicit speech from the child. Usually this requires discarding an assessment role in which we feel compelled to do something to or for the child. As experienced clinicians know, demanding adults prompt few utterances from children except "No," "I don't want to," "I can't," "Naa," and the like.

The primary goal in collecting a free-speech sample is to record what is representative of the child's usual productive language. The term *representative* implies both reliability and validity. Repeated samples should be similar in content, and the behavior of interest—productive language performance in a communicative context—is what is in fact recorded. Several aspects of productive interaction affect whether the sample is representative. These factors include the nature of the interaction, the setting, the materials, the method of recording, the sample size, and the context. Each of these aspects is discussed in turn as it relates to collecting a representative sample of the child's speech.

The Nature of the Interaction

Usually we think of interactions for the purpose of collecting free-speech samples only between clinician and child. It is important and often necessary to broaden this view. In our experience, many young children, particularly children between the ages of 9 and 30 months, have difficulty separating from their mothers. Other children do not relate well to strangers and simply refuse to talk to them. An alternative for these children is to record mother-child interactions. This can be accomplished by simply instructing the mother that "We want to see what Jim usually does; so please play with him as you would at home." A second alternative is to record child-child interactions, including playmates or siblings. If at all possible, try to secure part of the sample with the clinician and part with the mother. This provides the opportunity to analyze the mother's speech to the child, as well as to look for differences in the child's speech to different conversational partners.

With any interaction pair the clinician must monitor the communication exchange. Spontaneous interactions that maintain the child's interest and enthusiasm are the goal. When interacting with the child it is best for the adult to be interested without being pushy. Asking questions, particularly those to which the child knows the answer, and giving commands should be kept to a minimum. Asking open-ended questions such as "Tell me more," "What happened?," and "What's next?" can often get the child talking. It is helpful to remember that answers to questions are respondent behaviors that often take the form of sentence fragments and cannot be analyzed with many systems that require spontaneous, child-initiated utterances. Repeating what the child says will be helpful when the time comes for transcribing, particularly for children with poor intelligibility.

Children must be comfortable with the clinician before they will talk. But in addition to being friendly, warm, and interested, the clinician must adapt to the child's level of development in the conversation. Listening to the child, being patient, allowing some warm-up time to adapt to the child's performance level adds to the quality of the speech sample. And the complexity of the speech directed to the child should be attuned to his or her ability to comprehend. In order for children to engage in a conversation, they must understand what is being said to them. So, the clinician must monitor his or her speech, keeping within the child's comprehension repertoire. And since children's utterance frequency is very low up to 18 months, and continues to increase gradually to the adult rate, children cannot be expected to respond to speech addressed to them as consistently as adults would.

The most difficult part of collecting a representative free-speech sample is the beginning of the interaction, the "How do I get this child to talk to me?" problem. We have found the following strategies to be helpful in getting started:

1. *Saying nothing beyond initial friendly greetings for the first 5 minutes* This approach is particularly effective with children who are recalcitrant or self-conscious about their speech.
2. *Parallel play with little talking during the first few minutes* Any talking done is directed at toys rather than the child. This approach is effective with young children functioning at 30 months or below on cognitive tasks.
3. *Interactive play with little talking during the first few minutes* Toys can be shared by simply announcing, "I'm going to play with my gas station. You can play with it, too." There is no need to ask if the child wants to play, since he or she will likely say no. This approach is effective with children of cognitive level 3 to 5 years.
4. *Interactive play without an introduction* The clinician and child can work together drawing pictures or molding playdough. Participation and discussion can be invited after the activity is completed.

Note that these activities generally reflect developmental characteristics and will have to be modified to meet the child's perceptual, visual-auditory, and motor capabilities.

Setting

Samples can be collected in a number of settings.

1. Home—during various activities such as meals, dressing, playing.
2. School—classroom, therapy room or playground during various activities such as reading, instruction, group games, etc.
3. Residential facility—day room, ward, school room, therapy room during daily activities.
4. Clinic—waiting room, therapy room.

Representative samples can be collected almost anywhere, if the behavior of the adults in the conversation and the potential constraints the setting places on the child's behavior are monitored. The classroom, for example, may elicit only certain kinds of speech depending upon the activity: questions during worktime, and descriptions during show and tell. In some homes children are taught not to talk during mealtime. Each situation must be evaluated for potential constraints before collecting a sample. And if several children are being compared, attempts should be made to collect their speech samples under the same conditions.

In our experience, samples collected at the Waisman Center have been very representative.

Materials

The materials used in collecting speech samples should function as props to focus conversation, not as a substitute for interaction with the child. Materials should be selected for individual children according to cognitive level, interest, and auditory, visual, and motor functioning. The materials selected will constrain what the children talk about and how they talk about it. Discussing picture books tends to elicit routines, e.g., "Once upon a time, there were three bears (pigs, kittens, etc.)." Utterances learned as routines are not spontaneous. Games tend to evoke "It's your turn," counting, or a narrow set of questions ("Do you have the Old Maid?"). Puzzles do not require talking at all, or may serve to elicit locative vocabulary. We have found that toys that allow the child to construct a variety of activities elicit the most spontaneous speech from children up through Piaget's late preoperational period, or 6–7 years. Eating utensils, dolls, barns with appropriate animals, gas station with cars, people, and the Fisher-Price school house, school bus, castle, and house are excellent. They provide both familiar and unfamiliar materials. Many children have one or more of these toys, but usually the clinic has something the child does not have. We have found that children usually talk more about new and unique toys. If it is possible, ask the parent before the session what the child likes to play with; the answer will provide some direction in selecting materials.

Materials can be either presented to the child or set out for the child to discover. The first alternative, in which the clinician controls the choice, will provide consistency among evaluations, but it assumes that children are equally interested in all the materials used. The second option maximizes the child's interest, since children can choose to play with toys that have the most appeal for them. In our experience, the latter situation works best for children up to Piaget's concrete operational levels (7–8 years). In either case, moving materials off the table and onto the floor puts the adult at the child's level, makes the session less formal, and makes the child more comfortable.

In general, we have found that the more structured the interaction the less varied is the language used, in terms of both constructions and meanings expressed. Mean length of utterance (MLU), however, may be less affected by the structure imposed upon the session than are other measures. The implication is that if MLU is the only analysis procedure we perform, we may fail to observe differences in language production related to the setting, the materials, or the person interacting with the child.

In order to summarize the clinician's role in securing a representative sample of the child's speech, we have constructed a set of simple suggestions for engaging children in conversation and a set of principles to ensure conversational variety. This summary serves as a reminder of the clinician's role in gathering representative speech samples (see Tables 1 and 2).

Methods of Recording

Methods of recording what children say have included audiotaping, videotaping, or writing down the interaction. With both mechanical recording equipment and handwritten procedures, the goal is to reproduce faithfully what the child says. Some suggestions for implementing audio, video, and handwritten procedures are given below.

Audiotape Recordings

1. A good quality tape recorder and microphone, preferably with automatic gain control, is essential for accurate transcription.

2. Cassette recorders are much easier to handle than reel-to-reel machines.
3. Multidirectional microphones placed in close proximity to the child (1–3 feet) are preferred over tie-tack or lavalier microphones if the cord will constrain movement. FM microphones work exceptionally well if available.
4. Recorders may inhibit the children at first. The best procedure is to show children the equipment and let them get used to it, usually about 5 minutes, before beginning to record.
5. Making notes on the child's activities (what the child is playing with, what the child is doing) will aid transcription and provide information on nonverbal context that may not be evident from the audiotape alone.
   Note: You will not remember as much as you think you will.

Videotape Recordings

1. Suggestions 1–5 for audiotape recording are also applicable for videotape recordings.
2. The audio signal in video equipment is not always of sufficient quality to allow accurate transcription, particularly for phonological analysis. The simultaneous use of a high quality tape recorder with the videotaping results in the best audio reproduction as well as context.
3. Cameras can be very distracting. If taping through one-way glass is not possible, an adaptation period should be built into the session.

On-Line Transcription Procedures In certain situations when immediate results are needed or recording equipment is unavailable or impractical to use, the on-line, or as-it-happens, transcription procedure is the only alternative. Two aspects of verbal production determine the general approach and method used to record what the child says:

1. *The child's frequency of verbal production* It is difficult, if not impossible, to write down everything said by highly vocal children over a lengthy observation period.
2. *Dimensions of verbal production of interest: Phonology, syntax, semantics, or language functions* Phonological analysis requires the use of phonetic transcription. Syntactic or semantic analyses may require the child's utterance as well as notes on the context. Analyses of language functions require the child's utterance, adult or child utterances preceding and following the target utterance, and context notes.

Two general approaches to on-line transcription have been used. The first is simply to *write down everything* the child says relevant to the language di-

Table 1. Suggestions for conversations with children

1. **Listen**
   Focus on what the child means by what he or she says so your responses evidence shared focus.
2. **Be Patient**
   Do not overpower the child with requests or actions. Allow the child space and time to perform. Do not be afraid of pauses.
3. **Follow The Child's Lead**
   Maintain the child's focus (topic, meaning) with your responses, comments, questions, and add new information where appropriate. Maintain the child's pace, do not rush on to the next activity.
4. **Value The Child**
   Recognize the child's comments as important and worth your undivided attention. Do not patronize the child. Demonstrate unconditional positive regard. Be warm and friendly.
5. **Do Not Play The Fool**
   A valued conversational partner has something to say worth listening to. Refrain from asking questions that the child knows you know the answer to, or from making the usual remarks children hear from adults.
6. **Learn To Think Like A Child**
   Consider the child's perspective at different levels of cognitive development, and the child's awareness of the varying perspectives of action, time, and space.

Table 2. Getting children to talk about a variety of objects, events, and relationships

Linguistic stage (Brown, 1973)	Activities and materials
Pre-Stage I–Stage III	**Conversation** Make both familiar and unfamiliar toys available to the child. Include several examples of each class: balls, dolls, cups-glasses, cars, trucks.
Stage III–on	**Conversation** Introduce topics about absent objects, people, pets, and events displaced in time and space, e.g., holidays, vacations, school activities, grandma, child's room, favorite toys.
Stage IV–on	**Narration** In addition to conversation, prompt the child into narration on a topic displaced in time and space, e.g., telling a story about a past or future activity.

mensions of interest. In young children or children with limited verbal production, this procedure works quite well and maximizes the size of the corpus in the observation session.

The second approach is *time sampling*, in which the observer records what the child says for a limited time period through the assessment or observation session. For example, with highly verbal children or children in whom multiple production dimensions are to be evaluated, the clinician can transcribe for 1 to 5 minutes and rest for 1 to 5 minutes over a lengthy assessment or observation session. This procedure allows the clinician to shift dimensions in recording and maximizes his or her attention and the consistency of the transcripts. These time samples will usually cover a range of contexts and provide a more reliable transcript than one made in a single 10-to 15-minute on-line recording session.

There are two things to keep in mind when attempting on-line transcription. First, it gets easier with practice. We find high reliability for MLU analyses between on-line transcription and transcription from tapes for experienced clinicians (approximately 0.80 for MLU in morphemes). Second, setting up the transcription format before beginning will standardize recording and improve accuracy.

Sample Size

Two approaches can be taken in determining sample size. The first is simply to specify the number of child utterances at 50, 100, or 200 utterances. The second is to record for a specific period of time. We have found the latter approach to have a number of advantages over specifying the number of utterances. The major advantage is flexibility. Usually we only have so much time to spend with each child, and young children fatigue rather rapidly. In our experience, 30 minutes of interaction usually produces from 100 to 200 utterances in children functioning at 24 months of age and above. The 30 minutes fits our clinical schedule and most children can perform without fatigue for this period of time. This finding is confirmed by Crystal, Fletcher, and Garman (1976). For children functioning below 24 months of age fewer than 100 utterances can be expected. Between 18 and 24 months, about 30 to 60 utterances are produced in 30 minutes. Between 12 and 18 months, samples should be supplemented with daily logs kept by parents.

We divide these 30 minutes into two 15-minute play sessions, one with the mother and child and the other with the clinician and child. We transcribe every utterance for the 30-minute period, both adult's and child's. In order to get the best view of what the child is doing productively it is important not to discard utterances. The transcript can be segmented later for the types of utterances required to perform specific analyses like Developmental Sentence Scoring (DSS) (Lee, 1974), Language Sampling, Analysis, and Training (LSAT) (Tyack and Gottsleben, 1974), Linguistic Analysis of Speech Samples (LASS) (Engler, Hannah, and Longhurst, 1973), Indian Scale of Clausal Development (ISCD) (Dever and Bauman, 1974), Co-occurring and Restricted Structure Procedure (CORS) (Muma, 1973), or Language Assessment, Remediation, and Screening Procedure (LARSP) (Crystal et al., 1976). The transcript should include an indication of unintelligible utterances, with the number of syllables noted when possible. Imitations, false starts, hesitations, incomplete sentences, and answers to questions all have potential clinical value even though they cannot be directly analyzed by the procedures listed above. With a transcript that includes everything the child and the adult said for 30 minutes we have the flexibility to perform several kinds of analyses, the choice of which will depend upon our specific goals for the assessment.

The time sample format makes frequency analysis meaningful. There are a number of children, particularly retarded children, whose language structure and content are appropriate but who just do not talk very much. With time-restricted sampling procedures, this judgment can be substantiated.

In addition to the free-speech sample, we also collect and transcribe an additional 15-minute sample in which the clinician gives a variety of questions and commands. This sample provides the opportunity to analyze the children's comprehension through answers to questions and responses to commands. It also provides an opportunity to observe differences in the children's utterances when they are directed to respond in specific ways, rather than allowed to speak spontaneously. Specific elicitation procedures are discussed in Chapters 5 and 6.

Regardless of the method of recording used, the operating principle should be: If you are spending the time to transcribe the child's speech, do it right. Any analysis is only as good as the transcript on which it is based.

Context

The necessity of making contextual notes while collecting free-speech samples for syntactic and semantic analysis was demonstrated by Bloom (1970). Taking notes on what is happening while the child is talking has become standard practice and is considered essential for interpreting children's utterances.

The term *context* generally refers to the objects and events that precede, follow, or co-occur with the child's speech. Context, then, includes linguistic events (adult's speech, child's speech) as well as objects used, actions performed on objects, gestures, facial expressions, and visual line of regard observed during the interaction.

A record of the utterances the child heard before he or she responded is necessary in order to determine whether the child's utterance is an imitation or an answer to a question. A record of the child's or adult's behavior is necessary to interpret intended meaning of children's utterances, particularly in the one- to three-word stages. Bloom's (1970) classic example of the utterance "Mommy sock" illustrates this point: when uttered while the child is holding his or her mother's sock, it expresses a possessive relationship. If the child is holding his or her own sock, we infer an agent-object request ("Mommy, put on my sock"). Notes on objects present are particularly necessary for interpreting pronominal forms ("Where is it"?)

Inclusion of all adult and child utterances in the transcript ensures that linguistic context has been recorded. Objects present and child or adult actions can be recorded in a separate column adjacent to the utterance column.

An alternative to writing contextual notes adjacent to utterances is to gloss each utterance using all available context. For example: "He has it," He [Jim] has [is holding] it [ball]. This can be done at the time of or subsequent to the interaction using notes and tape recordings. This glossing procedure combines context and utterance to specify as precisely as possible the structure and meaning of each utterance. It avoids the problem of interpreting general contextual notes in relation to each utterance in terms of sequence (e.g., Did the child speak first or act first?)

The necessity of specifying the context depends, of course, on both the analytic procedures to be used and the child's language level. No context is necessary for computing MLU, for example. The shorter the child's utterances, the more context will be necessary to interpret them. As the child's sentences encode more of the context through the use of longer and more complex utterances, fewer nonlinguistic events are necessary to interpret them. Decisions on amount and type of context to be recorded should then be based on 1) degree of specificity required for particular analyses, both for the present and for possible future uses of the transcript, and 2) developmental level of the child. It is only necessary to record information that will be needed for analysis purposes. But the transcript should be interpretable 2 months, 6 months, or 1 year after it was recorded by someone who did not observe the assessment session.

TRANSCRIPTION OF TAPES

What level of detail is required in the transcript when multiple analysis procedures are to be carried out? The answer to this question varies depending upon specific assessment goals and the child's level and frequency of production. The analysis procedures presented in this section require only a morphemic transcription in standard English orthography. Clearly, aspects of phonology are relevant to morphology and often deserve phonetic transcription. For example, analysis of noun and verb inflections where allomorphic variation is of interest requires phonetic transcription. In addition, Ingram (personal communication) argues that as many as 40% of the utterances in orthographic transcripts may be lost for subsequent analysis because they are unintelligible. Phonetic transcription documents speech characteristics that are consistent, resulting in fewer unintelligible utterances. The decision as to whether or not to transcribe phonetically must be made for each child individually. Structural and semantic elements to be analyzed and the level of analysis required to document the child's language performance play a part in this decision. Obviously, time considerations are important, too, in determining level of detail, since phonetic transcription is a very time-consuming procedure.

The general guidelines outlined below have proved helpful in maintaining consistency of orthographic transcription. They provide a flexible format that contains the necessary data for variety of lexical, structural, and semantic analysis procedures. (The first page of a sample transcript is presented in Table 3 to illustrate these guidelines in use. For a complete sample transcript, refer to Chapter 2, pages 47–54.)

I. All transcriptions should be written in standard English orthography, with unintelligible utterances noted by using the International Phonetic Alphabet (IPA). All vocal and verbal behavior occurring during each interaction should be transcribed. Pauses in conversation are noted with the appropriate symbol. Temporal order of events in the transcript is maintained by numbering speakers' utterances consecutively.

II. Utterance segmentation should be based on terminal intonation contour, rising or falling. Pauses greater than 2 seconds both within and between utterances should be coded to determine their distri-

Table 3. Sample Transcript

Name of child: Mark
Clinic number:
Chronological age: 6–8
Date of evaluation:
Examiners:

Child MLU: 2.50
Number of utterances: 53
Number of intelligible utterances: 52
Sources of transcription: Audiotape

Adult MLU:
1. Mother
2. Clinician
3.

Key:

C = Child	[ ]	Gloss or Contextual notes
E = Examiner	( )	Questionable Transcription
XXX = unintelligible	/ /	Phonetic Transcription
. . . = pause		

Situation variables:
Time of day: 1:30 p.m.
Setting: Waisman Center (Rm. 145)
Materials used: Blocks, puzzle, PAT pictures, DLM pictures, puppet
Length of interaction: 18 minutes
Participants/Type of interactions: 1. Clinician-child
2.
3.
4.

Pragmatics		Speaker		Utterance Number	Dialogue	Morpheme Count		Syntax	Semantics
Child	Adult					Child	Adult		
		C		1.	Hey, that Cookie Monster stands.				
			E	1.	That stands?				
				2.	It sure does.				
				3.	Mark, do you know who this is?				
		C		2.	Oscar.				
			E	4.	Is that Oscar?				
				5.	Or is that the Cookie Monster?				
		C		3.	Oscar.				
			E	6.	Oscar!				
		C		4.	Cookie Monster in there. [box]				
			E	7.	The Cookie Monster's in there?				
				8.	I thought this was the Cookie Monster?				
		C			[shakes head]				

butional characteristics within and between utterances for individual children. In general, 80% of the pauses greater than 2 seconds will occur between utterances.

III. Glossing can be used as a device for combining context and utterance to specify, as far as possible, the structure and meaning of each utterance. Specifically, pronominals and utterances that require context to be interpreted should be glossed if context is not recorded separately.

IV. Whenever possible the reliability of each transcript should be determined by having a second transcriber listen to the tape with the transcript, noting corrections and disagreements. Before coding for analysis, these corrections and disagreements should be resolved to ensure an accurate transcript.

V. Information to be recorded on the first page of the transcript can include:
   A. Source of transcription
      1. Videotape
      2. Audiotape
      3. On-line
   B. Situational variables
      1. Time of day (e.g., 3:30 p.m.)
      2. Setting (place of interaction)
      3. Materials used (e.g., pictures, objects, toys)
      4. Length of interaction (minutes)
      5. Participants/Type of interaction
         a. Mother-child with few instructions given to mother
         b. Clinician-child with no verbal initiation by the clinician
         c. Clinician-child with questioning/commands/verbal initiations by the clinician
         d. Other: (e.g., child-child, child-father)

         Note: A minimum of two different interactions is preferred. Each interaction should last for 15 minutes, or until the child has produced at least 50 utterances.
      6. Transcription format
         a. Sequence of utterances
            1) Under the "Speaker" column, indent the adult utterances five spaces. For example:

Speaker	Utterance Number	Dialogue
Child	1	
Adult	1	
Child	2	
Adult	2	
Child	3	

            2) Number the intelligible utterances of each speaker sequentially under the column headed "Utterance Number" (as in example above).
         b. Symbols for transcription
            1) [ ] Gloss or contextual notes
               For example:
               Child's utterance: Mommy sit.
               Gloss: Mommy [is] sit[ting].
               Child's utterance: it go
               Gloss: it [the car] go[es]
            2) ( ) Questionable transcription
            3) / / Phonetic transcription when needed
            4) XXX Unintelligible utterance

               Note: Give an estimate of the length of the unintelligible utterance by making one or more groupings of "X" to indicate each syllable, when possible, or "XX" to indicate word segmentation.
            5) . . . Pause (either between speakers, or within a speaker's utterance, or between utterances of the same speaker)
         c. Punctuation
            1) Use standard punctuation, placing punctuation marks outside slashes / /!, and inside glosses [!].
         d. Key for speaker identifications
            1) C = Child (client)
            2) M = Mother
            3) E = Examiner (clinician)
            4) F = Father
            5) A = Another adult
            6) Ch = Another child

DIARY PROCEDURES

The discussion so far has been directed toward observation and recording of children's conversations in order to obtain a sample of the child's spontaneous speech. However, parent diaries can also be quite useful for obtaining these samples in a number of situations. The first arises when the representativeness of recorded samples is questionable. Parents often report that the child's speech during evaluation was different than it is at home. The second situation is the case of young children up to about 2 years of age whose frequency of speech is quite low. Third, reviewing a sample of speech before evaluation can often help in selecting assessment tasks for more in-depth analysis and can provide a comparison with the sample collected in the clinic. The fourth situation, monitoring change for children in treatment programs, requires documenting performance outside the treatment context to ensure generalization of learning. The use of diaries in any of these situations requires careful consideration of parent's ability to record representative samples.

We might ask who is the best judge of representativeness of the child's productive speech. Most of us would agree that the parents are, of course. They have spent the most time with the child. They have listened to the child talk. They know the child best. But even though we may agree that the parents know the child's speech best, we may question the parent's ability to record accurately what the child says. Our job is to supply parents with methods that allow them to make their knowledge explicit. We have found the diary a useful procedure for parents with sufficient time and interest to participate in their child's communicative assessment.

The diary format we have used with very young children can be found in the chapter appendix, on page 18. Using it requires us to specify carefully to parents the language behaviors of interest. These might include intentional communicative attempts, words, or sentences; specific sentence types, such as Wh-questions or negatives; and utterances produced in specific contexts, such as play with dad or siblings, and eating. Targets are determined by the assessment goals. Some training of parents will be necessary, and the more specific the target, the more training is required. With our general sampling procedures for young children, we have found that very little specific instruction is required other than what is given in the diary booklet itself. When problems arise, reviewing the diary with parents is the most effective training device. Significant improvement is observed with practice.

In some situations diaries may be the primary means of documenting performance status. For example, nonverbal children or those with severe motor impairments may initiate communicative attempts differently than other children do. Wants and needs may be expressed through body posture, visual line of regard, or gesture. These behaviors would be difficult to identify without spending considerable time with the child.

The diary format provides the mechanism for parents to make their knowledge of their child's communicative status explicit. We have found the diary to be a useful means of expanding and clarifying assessment data and securing parent participation in treatment. A set of diary-keeping instructions and a sample page are provided in the chapter appendix.

APPENDIX

DIARY OF COMMUNICATIVE DEVELOPMENT
Procedures for Parents

The purpose of the diary you are being asked to keep is to develop an accurate record of your child's communication development. This record is necessary because the communicative skills that your child displayed in our playroom may not be representative of what your child usually says. Specifically, we are interested in determining 1) the sounds and words that your child produces; 2) whether or not your child's sounds and words are imitations (did your child attempt to say all or a portion of what you had said immediately prior to his utterance); 3) whether or not your child's words are addressed to another, and, if so, to whom; 4) why your child said the word; and 5) what is happening in your child's immediate surroundings when the word is produced.

WHEN TO KEEP A DIARY

It has been our experience that if accurate records are carefully made during one day, a representative sample of your child's communicative behavior is obtained. Specifically, we recommend that records be kept during several activities on the day of observation. These activities include: 1) bathing, 2) diapering, 3) feeding, and 4) grooming. We ask that you choose any three periods during the day for observation. Additionally, you may choose an activity that you feel might be more representative of your child's communicative behavior.

HOW MUCH TIME WILL DIARY KEEPING TAKE?

Total diary observation and recording time should consume no more than 2 hours. Each situation (diapering, bathing, etc.) should yield between 15–20 minutes of observation. Of this time, only 10–15 minutes will be required for recording above and beyond the time you would normally be spending with your child.

HOW ARE DIARY RECORDS KEPT?

We have provided forms that specify the information you are to record. A sample form is provided at the end of these instructions. It is probably most convenient to have a diary page at each location in which you will be observing your child. Information should be placed in the diary as often as possible during the observational period. If you did not have an opportunity for on-going note-taking, it is desirable to take 5 to 10 minutes at the conclusion of the observational periods and fill in the relevant information.

WHAT IS TO BE RECORDED IN THE DIARY?

We are interested in determining the sounds and words that your child uses even though the words may not be completely intelligible. It is important that we have information on the child's typical vocabulary. Obtaining records of the child's words at home will help us to understand words he produced in our playroom. It is entirely possible that many of your child's words may be understandable to you, but not to an observer who doesn't see the child often. Examples of diary word entries are found below.

Word Produced	***Word Meant***
boat	boat
baba	boat
ma ma	milk
ga	?

It is also important that you write down sounds your child produces (as accurately as possible). In the last example the child produces "ga." The parent did not know what the child meant. Consequently, there is no entry under the category of "word meant."

WAS THE CHILD'S WORD(S) IMITATED?

If your child imitates a word that you have just said, we cannot be sure that this particular word occurs naturally in your child's repertoire.

Example:

Mother	***Child***	
car	car	Imitative child speech
There's a boat there	water	

DID THE CHILD DIRECT WORD(S) TO ANOTHER?

We know that children at very early ages direct words to mothers, fathers, and siblings. We also know that some words may be uttered without being specifically directed to another. We are interested in discovering both words used in communicating with others and words that are not directed to others.

WHAT WAS HAPPENING AND WHO WAS PRESENT WHEN THE WORD WAS PRODUCED?

To help us better understand the possible ways in which children learn to produce words it is essential that we know the specific components of the interactive setting. These include 1) objects within reach of your child, 2) people in the immediate area, 3) activity of the people in the immediate area, and 4) your child's activity.

WHY DID YOUR CHILD PRODUCE THE WORD?

This category is useful in helping us determine the reason for your child's saying a word. For example, if your child says *bottle,* gets no response from the adult and proceeds to cry, it is probable that your child said the word because he or she wanted the bottle. It is important to write the reason your child uttered the word only when you are *not* guessing at the reason (see the sample diary for examples).

All diary information will be kept confidential. Copies will be made available if you would like to include your diary in your child's baby book.

Sample Diary

Child's Name ______________________

Date ______________________

Observation began ______________________

Ended ______________________

Activity ______________________

Word meant	Word said	Imitated?	Spoken to someone?	Why child said it	Describe what was happening
dark	a (as in *at*)	no	M	C looked out window at night & saw it was dark	C & M in living room at night
pacifier	ba	no	M	C wanted his pacifier	C getting ready to go to bed
sock	o (as in *hot*)	no	F	C wanted father to put on his socks	C came in from outside with F
bath	ba	no	M	C wanted a bath	C came in from outside and was dirty
flower	owm	yes	M & F	C was picking flowers	M, F, & C talking about flowers
bike	bi	no	M	C wanted to take bike outside	C & M getting ready to go outside
sugar	sugar (mouthed)	no	M	C wanted some sugar	C eating a bowl of cereal
turn	ur	no	NO	C saw person on TV turned around	C watching TV
mama	mama	no	M	C wanted M to put shoes on	C & M getting ready to go away

CHAPTER 2

Procedures for Analyzing Free-Speech Samples: *Syntax and Semantics*

Contents

The aim of this chapter is to outline specific procedures for using free-speech sample analysis to describe children's productive language. Two kinds of procedures are included: 1) procedures for quantifying structural and semantic development to determine the child's developmental status, and 2) procedures for analyzing structural or semantic problem areas. The procedures included are not intended to be exhaustive, but they represent levels of analysis we have found useful. They are to be seen as guidelines and should be adapted to the clinician's own style, work situation, and time limits. Most important, they should be adapted specifically for each child being served.

The major criteria for the inclusion of procedures in this section are: 1) they have been clinically useful during our 7 years of experience at the Waisman Center on Mental Retardation and Human Development, 2) there are normative developmental data that relate to the results of the procedure, and 3) the procedures provide descriptions of productive language development that can be used to develop individualized intervention programs. Other procedures already available in the clinical literature are summarized in Tables 1 and 7.

Where possible, interpretive developmental data are included with each procedure. These data should be used as rough guidelines for establishing appropriate expectations, but not as hard-and-fast rules. The inherent variability of productive language development, the relatively few children studied in detail thus far, and our general state of knowledge about children's language development would make the assignment of specific ages, rather than age ranges, inappropriate and premature. On the other hand, it would be incorrect to ignore the normal developmental data, limited though they are, in favor of theoretical or clinical "hunches" as to the status of the child's productive syntax and semantics.

An old adage says that "practice makes perfect." This wisdom is particularly appropriate for developing our own skills in analyzing free-speech samples. Practice with these procedures will perfect our ability to make *informed* clinical judgments—before, one hopes, we achieve the status of grandparents ourselves.

GENERAL ANALYSES

The analysis of a transcript can take a number of different directions, depending upon the assessment goals set for the child. After transcribing the adult-child conversation, the clinician usually has a good notion of the child's general productive abilities. Specific analytic procedures should be selected to quantify those intuitions, to provide documentation, and to allow comparisons from child to child. We have found it helpful to first carry out some general analyses that quantify the entire sample. Such quantification provides a broad view of the child's performance and helps to identify specific problems requiring subsequent detailed analysis.

A number of procedures have been developed to provide general indices of various linguistic elements for an entire sample. Table 1 lists some of these procedures, the linguistic elements quantified, sample size advised, and age range of use. Of the procedures given in Table 1, the ones we have found particularly useful with our clinical population of developmentally disabled children include computing mean length of utterance (MLU) in words or morphemes for the child and the adult, and distributional analysis summarizing the number of one-, two-, three-, four-, etc., word utterances the child and the adult each produce. The MLU measures provide an index of syntactic complexity in the child's speech at least up to Stage V (MLU in morphemes= 4.0, Brown, 1973). The adult MLU provides an index of the complexity of speech directed to the child. The distributional analysis provides a view of the variety of utterance lengths contributing to MLU. A variety of sentence lengths is to be expected. When this variety is not found, additional diagnostic work is indicated. For example, children with MLUs of 2.0 are usually producing a number of one-word utterances as well as three-, four-, and a few five- and six-word utterances. A child producing almost entirely two-word utterances (e.g., 145 of 160) would be unusual and we would want to ask why the child's utterance length is so limited. Respiratory control for speech might be questioned, as would the degree to which the speech sample consisted of answers to *What's that?* questions.

A measure that is useful in quantifying general semantic aspects of the sample is the type-token ratio (TTR). This procedure is discussed in more detail in the section on semantic analyses. It provides a view of vocabulary diversity that is useful to compute when vocabulary is in question, or when a very general index of semantic development is needed.

Computing Mean Length of Utterance in Morphemes

by Robin S. Chapman

After segmenting the child's speech into utterances using the criterion of terminal intonation contour, rising or falling, mean length of utterance (MLU) measures can be computed for each speaker. The following procedures are adapted from Brown (1973, p. 54). They differ from his in using only 50, rather than 100, utterances and in failing to omit the first pages of the transcript.

Table 1. **General analysis procedures for quantifying transcripts of free-speech samples**

Content	Measure	Sample size advised	Range of use	Reference
Syntax	Mean Length of Utterance in Morphemes (MLU)	50 utterances or more	1.5–5 years	Brown, 1973; this volume;
	Mean Length of Utterance in Words (MLR)	50 utterances	1.5–8 years	Templin, 1957
	Mean Length of T-unit or Communication Unit (MLTR)	30 T-units	5–18 years	Loban, 1976
	Frequency distribution—Number of utterances by length	50 utterances[a]	1.5–18 years	This volume
	Frequency distribution—Number of utterances by structural type	50 utterances[a]	1.5–18 years	This volume
	Developmental Sentence Score (DSS)	50 utterances or more	3–7 years	Lee, 1974
	Length-Complexity Index (LCI)	15–50 utterances	4–8 years	Shriner, 1967, 1969; Miner, 1969; Barlow and Miner, 1969; Griffith and Miner, 1969
Semantics	Type-Token Ratio–Vocabularity Diversity	50 utterances or more	3–8 years	Templin, 1957
Phonology	Percent intelligible, partially intelligible, and unintelligible utterances	50 utterances[a]	1–18 years	
Communicative interaction	Frequency distribution of number of utterances per speaking turn for each speaker,	50 utterances[a]		
		50 utterances[a]	1–18 years	
	Mom's MLU-Child's MLU ratio,	50 utterances[a]	1.5–5 years	Retherford, Schwartz, and Chapman, in press
	number of Mom's utterances to number of Child's utterances	50 utterances[a]	2–18 years	Retherford, Schwartz, and Chapman, in press

[a]Number of utterances may vary for these analysis procedures. Fifty utterances is considered a minimum target providing enough data for interpretation. Note that as sample size increases, representativeness is likely to increase.

Selecting the Utterances to Include in the Computation

1. Unintelligible or partially unintelligible utterances are omitted from the count, but transcriptions marked doubtful are included.
2. The morphemes in the first 50 consecutive utterances in the sample (including exact utterance repetitions) are counted.

Counting Morphemes in Each Utterance A morpheme is a minimal meaningful unit of a language: for example, *dog* or plural-*s*. For an adult's language we can guess what a morpheme is from our own knowledge of the language, but for a child we need to find evidence to support our guesses. Counting rules based on Brown (1973), listed below, give the morphemic decisions made for the children. These should be used to compute comparable MLUs. Total number of morphemes for each counted utterance on the transcript is recorded.

1. Stuttering is marked as repeated efforts at a single word; the word is counted once in the most complete form produced. In the few cases where a word is produced for emphasis, or the like (*no, no, no*), each occurrence is counted separately.
2. Such fillers as *mm* or *oh* are not counted, but *no, yeah,* and *hi* are.
3. All compound words (two or more free morphemes), proper names, and ritualized reduplications count as single words. Some examples are *birthday, rackety-boom, choo-choo, quack-quack, night-night, pocketbook, see saw.* The justification for this decision is that there is no evidence that the constituent morphemes function as such for these children.
4. All irregular pasts of the verb (*got, did, went, saw*) count as one morpheme. Again, there is no evidence that the child relates these to present form.
5. All diminutives (*doggie, mommie*) count as one morpheme because these children do not seem to use the suffix productively. Diminutives are the standard forms used by the child.
6. All auxiliaries (*is, have, will, can, must, would*) count as separate morphemes as do all catenatives (*gonna, wanna, hafta, gotta*). The catenatives are counted as single morphemes, rather than as *going to* or *want to,* because evidence is that they function as such for children. All inflections, for example, possessive (*s*), plural (*s*), third person singular (*s*), regular past (*ed*), and progressive (*ing*), count as separate morphemes.

Computing MLU To compute MLU we first find the total number of morphemes for the speaker, then divide by the total number of utterances counted. The result is the MLU in morphemes.

Checking on the Representativeness of MLU We generally check transcripts for the following characteristics, any one of which may affect the obtained MLU. (Familiarity of listener, setting, and topic are, of course, other factors to likely affect MLU.)

1. *High rate of imitation of the previous speaker (e.g., exceeding 20% of child's utterances)* If the child imitates the other person's speech frequently, we would ask whether MLU is being increased unrepresentatively beyond the child's usual utterance length of spontaneous utterances. The simple thing to do is to compute MLU separately for the spontaneous utterances. If it is markedly shorter or longer (e.g., a linguistic stage) than the MLU for the total sample, it may be necessary to consider analyzing the imitative and spontaneous utterances separately. In that case, we would report not only total MLU, but MLU computed for each kind of utterance.
2. *Frequent self-repetitions within a speech turn* Brown includes self-repetitions in MLU counts; Bloom (1970, 1973) excludes them. If these utterances occur frequently in a transcript and are shorter, or longer, than most utterances, the decision to include them may bias the MLU value. Again, the simple procedure is to count MLU both ways and see whether it makes a difference of at least a stage (0.5 MLU). If it does, MLU values both including and excluding self-repetitions should be reported. In either case, structural analysis of an extended 50-utterance sample that excludes self-repetitions can be carried out to increase the variety of structural types available for inspection in the sample.
3. *High proportion of question-answers in the child's speech* If the child has been bombarded by questions we may expect to find reduced spontaneous speech and MLUs shorter than those characteristic of spontaneous utterances. This is because most questions are properly answered not by complete sentences but by parts of them ("There," "Yes," "No," "Looking"). Most samples of mother-child conversation contain a number of requests for information—indeed, such requests may typically make up more than one-third of the mother's utterances to children beginning to put two words together (Folger and Chapman, 1978). To exclude the child's

answers to questions entirely, then, would be to make it impossible to compare the sample directly to Brown's data which we would like to be able to do in order to assign the sample to one of Brown's stages. However, if the ratio of questions to the child exceeds 30%–40% of the adult's utterances, it may be necessary to ask whether the sample is representative of the other speaker's behavior or simply indicative of a novice student's nervous first attempts to get a child to talk. Even if the interaction is typical of that speaker, it may be wise to obtain a second speech sample with another speaker so that you can evaluate the child's MLU and structures under less constraining conditions. Or, we can again resort to the option of computing two MLUs, one including responses to questions and one excluding them. If this choice is made, both scores can be reported, although stage assignment will have to be based on the MLU that follows Brown's procedure.

4. *Frequent routines (counting, alphabet, nursery rhymes, song fragments, commercial jingles or long utterances made up by listing objects in a book or the room)* If there are frequent longer (or shorter) utterances that are recitations based on memory or picture content, the MLU may be biased by the inclusion of these utterances. Again, the recommended procedure is to compute MLU in two ways, including and excluding these utterances, and to report both if the results differ. If it makes no difference, routines may still be excluded from, or compared with, an extended sample for structural analysis. Memorized routines in particular may not be characteristic of the child's spontaneous constructions.
5. *High proportion of utterances in which clauses are conjoined by **and*** In speech samples of MLU greater than 4.0 or 5.0, instances of sentence conjunction become increasingly frequent; indeed, elementary school children may begin every sentence of a narrative with *And then*. . . Clearly you do not want to credit such samples with MLUs of 30! A large number of such sentences, or MLUs computed greater than 5.0, may signal the need to turn to other utterance measures better designed to reflect increased grammatical sophistication in the child. The best of these appears to be the T-unit or communication unit (Loban, 1976) count. T-units ignore *and* conjoinings, and false starts or "garbles" in the child's utterances, and treat each clause headed by *and* as one unit of communication. The morphemes within this unit are counted, and the total number of units is used as the denominator in calculating mean length of T-unit.

Interpreting Mean Length of Utterance in Morphemes

When interpreting the significance of a child's MLU as a description or quantification of productive language status, several cautions must be kept in mind. First, MLU is to be used only as a general indicator of structural development, and it can only be reliably interpreted when it falls between 1.01 and 4.49 (Brown, 1973). It is not a substitute or a replacement for more detailed structural analysis. The second caution is that MLU can only be interpreted when the criteria for representativeness of the speech sample have been satisfied. Samples should be reviewed for spontaneity of conversation, potential constraints of the setting, materials, recording procedure, sample size, and context, and for the specific characteristics detailed in the previous section by Chapman. *Remembering that MLU is only an index and that we must guarantee the representativeness of the sample from which it is derived will help prevent its overinterpretation.*

Stage of Structural Development Brown and his colleagues studied speech samples that were as close as possible in MLU value to the target values 1.75, 2.25, 2.75, 3.5, and 4.0 in three children. It proved useful for describing structural development to divide the MLU continuum into ranges around these midpoints; these are Brown's Linguistic Stages I through V. De Villiers and de Villiers (1973a) have smoothed the original cuts to intervals of 0.5 morphemes, retaining Brown's labels of 1973 (see Table 2). Brown's stages are applicable only when the child has started to combine some words; that is, when MLU is greater than 1.00.

Each stage, although somewhat arbitrarily defined by MLU value, is associated with distinct developmental achievements and to this extent the stages can be said to be qualitatively different from one another (Morehead and Ingram, 1973; Morehead and Morehead, 1974).

The child's MLU defines his or her stage assignment in Brown's scheme. For example, an MLU of 2.70 places the child in Brown's Stage III, an MLU of 3.40 places the child in Early Stage IV. These stages define the structures we can expect to be present in the child's productive speech. A detailed account of the normal sequence of structural development by stage is found in the charts containing the

Table 2. Predicted chronological ages and age ranges within one standard deviation of the predicted value for each MLU

Brown's stage	MLU	Predicted chronological age[a]	Predicted age ± 1 SD[b] (middle 68%)
Early Stage I MLU = 1.01–1.49	1.01	19.1	16.4–21.8
	1.10	19.8	17.1–22.5
	1.20	20.6	17.9–23.3
	1.30	21.4	18.7–24.1
	1.40	22.2	19.5–24.9
	1.50	23.0	18.5–27.5
Late Stage I MLU = 1.50–1.99	1.60	23.8	19.3–28.3
	1.70	24.6	20.1–29.1
	1.80	25.3	20.8–29.8
	1.90	26.1	21.6–30.6
	2.00	26.9	21.5–32.3
Stage II MLU = 2.00–2.49	2.10	27.7	22.3–33.1
	2.20	28.5	23.1–33.9
	2.30	29.3	23.9–34.7
	2.40	30.1	24.7–35.5
	2.50	30.8	23.9–37.7
Stage III MLU = 2.50–2.99	2.60	31.6	24.7–38.5
	2.70	32.4	25.5–39.3
	2.80	33.2	26.3–40.1
	2.90	34.0	27.1–40.9
	3.00	34.8	28.0–41.6
Early Stage IV MLU = 3.00–3.49	3.10	35.6	28.8–42.4
	3.20	36.3	29.5–43.1
	3.30	37.1	30.3–43.9
	3.40	37.9	31.1–44.7
	3.50	38.7	30.8–46.6
Late Stage IV–Early Stage V MLU = 3.50–3.99	3.60	39.5	31.6–47.4
	3.70	40.3	32.4–48.2
	3.80	41.1	33.2–49.0
	3.90	41.8	33.9–49.7
	4.00	42.6	36.7–48.5
Late Stage V MLU = 4.00–4.49	4.10	43.4	37.5–49.3
	4.20	44.2	38.3–50.1
	4.30	45.0	39.1–50.9
	4.40	45.8	39.9–51.7
	4.50	46.6	40.3–52.9
Post Stage V MLU = 4.50 +	4.60	47.3	41.0–53.6
	4.70	48.2	41.9–54.5
	4.80	48.9	42.6–55.2
	4.90	49.7	43.4–56.0
	5.00	50.5	42.1–58.9
	5.10	51.3	42.9–59.7
	5.20	52.1	43.7–60.5
	5.30	52.8	44.4–61.2
	5.40	53.6	45.2–62.0
	5.50	54.4	46.0–62.8
	5.60	55.2	46.8–63.6
	5.70	56.0	47.6–64.4
	5.80	56.8	48.4–65.2
	5.90	57.5	49.1–65.9
	6.00	58.3	49.9–66.7

[a]Age is predicted from the equation Age (in months) = 11.199 + 7.857 (MLU)

[b]Computed from obtained standard deviations

criteria for Assigning Structural Stage (ASS) (chapter appendix B, pages 55–66). To the extent that MLU indexes structural achievements, the linguistic stage assignment provides a description of the structures the child has acquired or is in the process of acquiring. The child's MLU, then, shows generally where he or she is in the sequence of structural acquisition. In order to determine if the child's MLU is within expectation of the child's age we need to know the relationship between age and MLU.

Predicting Age from MLU Miller and Chapman (1979) investigated the relationship between age and MLU in 123 children, 17–59 months of age, in a Madison, Wisconsin community. Speech samples of at least 50 utterances were gathered in mother-child conversational contexts and MLUs in morphemes were computed using Brown's rules with a few modifications. Analysis reveals a strong correlation between age and MLU ($r=0.88$), with 77% of the variance accounted for. Standard deviations increased with age. In addition, regression analysis revealed that the relation between MLU and age was essentially linear, indicating that age and MLU change systematically with respect to each other in a manner best represented by a straight line. An equation can then be derived that describes the line of best fit for MLU regressed on age or age on MLU. In this way, age can be predicted given a calculated MLU, or MLU can be predicted given a specific age. The age and MLU predictions in Table 2 along with their standard deviations provide a means to interpret age-appropriateness of the MLU a child in a clinical population displays. Table 2 can be used to derive the predicted age for a calculated MLU by rounding off the calculated MLU to the nearest tenth and locating it on the table. For example, for an MLU of 2.20 an age of 28.5 months and an age range within one standard deviation (±1 SD) of 23–34 months is predicted. (The ±1 SD describes the performance range of 68% of any population.) Standard deviations were calculated for age at 3-month intervals (see Table 3) and for MLU at 0.10 MLU intervals (see Table 2). An MLU of 3.4 can be expected of 68% of the children between 31 and 45 months of age.

Our interest in the chronological age (CA)-MLU relationship is, of course, to help us to quantify our judgment of delayed productive language status. Specifically, we want to know whether the child's structural stage is appropriate to his or her CA, in addition to knowing what that stage is.

Considerable caution should be exercised in interpreting the CA-MLU relationship for an individual child. The data in Tables 2 and 3 should not be considered exhaustively normative. These data are from a reasonably small sample of middle-class children from Madison, Wisconson and are not necessarily representative of all children in the state of Wisconsin or any other state. We would expect the same significant relationship to be demonstrated with

Table 3. Predicted MLUs and MLU ranges within one standard deviation of predicted mean for each age group

Age ±1 Month	Predicted MLU[a]	Predicted SD[b]	Predicted MLU ±1 SD (middle 68%)
18	1.31	0.325	0.99-1.64
21	1.62	0.386	1.23-2.01
24	1.92	0.448	1.47-2.37
30	2.54	0.571	1.97-3.11
33	2.85	0.633	2.22-3.48
36	3.16	0.694	2.47-3.85
39	3.47	0.756	2.71-4.23
42	3.78	0.817	2.96-4.60
45	4.09	0.879	3.21-4.97
48	4.40	0.940	3.46-5.34
51	4.71	1.002	3.71-5.71
54	5.02	1.064	3.96-6.08
57	5.32	1.125	4.20-6.45
60	5.63	1.187	4.44-6.82

[a]MLU is predicted from the equation $MLU = -0.548 + 0.103\,(age)$.

[b]SD is predicted from the equation $SD_{MLU} = -0.0446 + 0.0205\,(age)$.

other populations of different socioeconomic status and geographic location, but the exact CAs and MLUs predicted may not be the same as those in Tables 2 and 3. Therefore, the CA predictions for a specific MLU should not be used as the only criteria for determining the presence of a developmental delay.

The Miller and Chapman study clearly shows that variability of MLU and CA increases with advancing CA and higher MLU. While we would not expect the exact figures in Tables 2 and 3 to be sustained for populations in different locales and socioeconomic groups, the predictions are clinically informative in a number of ways.

The socioeconomic status and educational level of the Madison community is generally middle to upper-middle class. As a result, we would expect the CA-MLU predictions from this sample of children to be on the high end of the distribution of these characteristics in the general population. Clinically, children performing within one standard deviation of the mean should clearly be within normal limits. Those at or below one standard deviation from the mean require further study with detailed analysis of their structural development, although the CA-MLU discrepancy itself is not sufficient evidence to diagnose a language delay. Tables 2 and 3, then, are useful in determining which children require further evaluation. This preliminary step in structural analysis allows us to spend more time analyzing the transcripts of children whose structural development is questionable.

While the relationship between mental age (MA) and MLU has not been specifically studied, data from a developmentally disabled population (Miller, Chapman, and Bedrosian, 1978) suggest as strong a correlation as that found between chronological age and MLU. Mean length of utterance in words appears highly related to MA in a comparison of gifted subjects (Fisher, 1934) and normal subjects (McCarthy, 1954) of the same chronological age. These studies imply that some form of the Cognition Hypothesis, which proposes that certain cognitive developments are prerequisites for language use, holds true for MLU as an index of general structural development. We have found it useful to derive the CA predictions for MLUs of retarded children and compare the predicted CAs with their mental age and other language measures, rather than with their chronological age. For these children, the CA predictions related to MA provide a good basis for comparison with various comprehension measures. Mental age, MA, then, appears to be a more valid metric for interpreting the language performance of retarded children than does chronological age (Miller, 1978). While explicit experimental confirmation of either the appropriate form of the Cognition Hypothesis, whether causal or correlational, or the MA-MLU relation in retarded populations is lacking, we find the CA-MLU data in Tables 2 and 3 clinically useful in determining the presence of language delay above and beyond the general cognitive retardation. We feel justified in using the MA-MLU relationship in this way since it is but one of several structural analysis procedures performed. However, as we have cautioned before, CA-MLU data are only used to explore comparisons among production variables and among production, comprehension, and mental age. *MLU should never be used alone as the basis for determining a child's structural development status.*

Distributional Analysis

A distributional analysis is a reorganization of the transcript by specific utterance characteristics. We have found segmentation of transcripts by sentence length, by syntactic structure, and by number of utterances per speaking turn to be useful. Specifically, distributional analysis by sentence length will help clarify MLU measures by quantifying the number of utterances produced at each length. Variation around the mean should exist, but a number of spuriously long utterances may inflate the MLU and render it unrepresentative. Speech samples with utterances of all the same length, particularly one or two words, may indicate a limitation in productive span due to functional problems in the speech mechanism.

Distributional analysis by syntactic structure provides a view of structural variety in the sample. It also serves as a first step in examining structural development in detail using the *Assigning Structural Stage* (ASS) procedure (chapter appendix B). This type of segmentation allows examination of the specific structures produced and the usual length of utterance with which they are associated. Structures produced within longer utterances or low frequency utterances may be in initial stages of acquisition.

Distributional analysis of the number of utterances per speaking turn looks at a more pragmatic level of productive language. In this analysis both child and adult utterances need to be segmented. The relationship between the number of utterances per speaking turn for the child and the adult reflects the distribution of talking in the sample for each speaker. This distribution may also reflect the child's turn-taking ability in conversation and the degree to which the adult allowed the child to talk.

There are no specific interpretive data for these analyses. They should all be considered initial procedures that can help identify specific problem areas warranting further examination. To help communicate the value of these procedures for evaluating productive language, each analysis was performed on the sample transcript in chapter appendix A, pages 47–54. Results of utterance length distribution are listed in Table 4, structural distribution in Table 5, and the distribution of utterances per speaking turn in Table 6.

The first step in interpreting MLU is to examine the distribution of utterance lengths in the sample. Utterance lengths should be distributed around the mean. Utterances that are one, two, or three morphemes longer and shorter than the mean are expected, depending upon the MLU value. For example, a speech sample with an MLU of 3.1 should include utterances of 4-, 5-, 6- and perhaps even some 7-morpheme utterances as well as utterances of 1 and 2 morphemes. If the distribution is constrained in any way we must ask why. A speech sample with an MLU of 2.0 that only contains utterances two morphemes long is cause for suspicion. We would want to ask what other constraints beyond linguistic competence could be limiting the child's production. Further evaluation in both speech motor control, particularly respiratory capacity, and input, would indicate the nature of the utterances directed to the child. Distributional analysis is also a good method of checking that the sample is not biased by utterances directed to the child that require short answers. *The distributional analysis must be done before MLU can be properly interpreted.*

SYNTACTIC ANALYSES

As we have seen, the computation of MLU and distributional analysis can be helpful in directing further analysis of the transcript. The child's syntactic stage of development as determined by MLU will orient our analysis for specific syntactic structures and semantic meanings. A set of general developmental expectations that can serve as a checklist can be derived for each stage based on MLU.

For example, for children performing in linguistic Stages I–III, who are producing predominantly simple sentences, a detailed analysis of semantics could involve computing a type-token ratio (page 42), and coding and summarizing the semantic roles

Table 4. Distribution of utterance lengths in sample transcript (chapter appendix A)

Number of morphemes per utterance	Child's utterance number from transcript	Total number of utterances
Utterances with 1 morpheme	2, 3, 7, 13, 15, 20, 23, 29, 30, 31, 32, 33, 34, 35, 42, 43, 46, 47, 48, 50	20
Utterances with 2 morphemes	5, 25, 39, 41	4
Utterances with 3 morphemes	4, 6, 10, 11, 14, 16, 17, 19, 21, 22, 26, 27, 28, 37, 40, 49, 52	17
Utterances with 4 morphemes	8, 9, 12, 18, 24, 36, 45, 50	8
Utterances with 5 morphemes	1	1
Utterances with 6 morphemes	44	1
Utterances with 7 morphemes		0
Utterances with 8 morphemes	38	1

Table 5. Distribution of simple sentence structures in sample transcript (chapter appendix A)

Structural analysis	Child's utterance number from transcript	Total number of utterances
Noun phrase elaboration	1, 4, 28, 38, 44, 45,	6
Verb phrase elaboration	8, 9, 16, 19, 21, 22, 36, 38, 44, 50, 52	11
Noun inflections	49	1
Verb inflections	1	1
Yes/no questions	6, 8, 9, 14, 17, 18, 24, 26, 27, 38, 45, 51	12
Wh-questions	19, 21, 22, 36, 50	5
Negation		0

expressed in the child's sentences (see section on Semantic analyses for details). Analysis of syntax for these children might focus on the first 7 of Brown's 14 morphemes, and noun phrase and verb phrase elaboration in simple sentences. For children performing in linguistic Stages IV and V, further semantic analysis could include semantic role analysis of simple sentences, semantic field analysis, and sentence conjunctions (Clancy, Jacobsen, and Silva, 1976). Syntactic analysis for children in Stages IV and V would examine the last 7 of the 14 grammatical morphemes, auxiliary structures, yes/no questions, Wh-questions, negation, and sentence embedding and sentence conjoining characteristics of complex sentences. Procedures for in-depth analysis of free-speech samples including recommended sample size and age range are listed in Table 7.

One of the difficult and frustrating aspects of syntactic analysis is describing the developmental relationship between various sentence structures seen from Stage I through Stage V. For example, auxiliary verb development in simple, active affirmative declarative sentences can be described. But this description does not capture the role that auxiliary verbs play in the development of yes/no questions, Wh-questions, or negation. Auxiliary development requires separate description in each of these structures. Such a set of descriptions is necessary in order to examine the development of sentence types in which the auxiliary plays a primary role. For example, a child with auxiliaries present in affirmative declarative sentences (at least Stage IV) may omit them in yes/no questions (Stage III or earlier). Or a child with Stage V auxiliary development in affirmative declarative sentences may neither prepose the auxiliary in yes/no questions *(I can ride it?)* nor invert the auxiliary in Wh-questions *(What he can ride in?)*.

Table 6. Distribution of number of utterances per speaking turn for child and adult in sample transcript (chapter appendix A)

	Utterances per turn					
Speaker	1	2	3	4	5	18
Child	51	3	0	0	0	0
Adult	28	14	5	5	1	1

The structural analysis procedure we have developed provides for comparison across structures. The child's transcript is segmented into major structural categories: the 14 grammatical morphemes, active affirmative declarative sentences, negatives, yes/no questions, Wh-questions, and complex sentences including embedding and conjoining. The level of development for each of these categories is determined by comparing the instances of each category in the transcript with the normal sequence of structural development charts containing the criteria for Assigning Structural Stage (chapter appendix B). Six types of structural development are analyzed: Production in the Single-Word Utterance Period (I), Noun Phrase Elaboration (II), Verb Phrase Elaboration (III), Negation (IV), Yes/No Questions (V), and Wh-Questions (VI). For example, active affirmative declarative sentences would be analyzed for noun phrase elaboration, verb phrase elaboration, and auxiliary development. The structural development charts provide the data necessary to determine a developmental stage for each structural component. The pattern of developmental stages that results provides an overview of structural development as well as the specific structural description necessary to construct a teaching program when necessary.

Except for the 14 grammatical morphemes, the data contained in the structural development charts show the stage at which research literature indicates each structure first appears in child speech. Unless otherwise noted, the charts list the stage at which structures emerge, not the stage at which they are mastered. Because the charts are drawn from a variety of studies, the criteria for emergence are not always the same. Chapman, Paul, and Wanska's (in preparation) criterion for emergence was the use of a structure at least once in a fifteen-minute speech sample by 50% of the children within an MLU group-

Table 7. Procedures for in-depth analysis of children's free-speech samples

Content	Procedure	Sample size	Range of use	Reference
Syntax	Developmental Sentence Types (DST)	100 utterances	22 months–6 years	Lee, 1966
	Developmental Sentence Analysis (DSS)	50 complete sentences	3–7 years	Lee, 1974
	Language Sampling, Analysis and Training (LSAT)	100 utterances	2–10 years[a]	Tyack and Gottsleben, 1974
	Language Assessment, Remediation and Screening Procedure (LARSP)	30 minutes 100–200 utterances	22 months–5 years[a]	Crystal, Fletcher, and Garman, 1976
	Scale of Children's Clausal Development (SCCD)	Transcript of unspecified length	18–40 months	Dever and Bauman, 1974
	TALK-Assessing Current Functioning	6–8 pages (200 + utterances)	1.5–5 years[a]	Dever, 1978
	Co-occurring and Restricted Structure Procedure (CORS)	Representative sample (usually requiring several samples in varying situations)	1.5–5 years[a]	Muma, 1973
	Linguistic Analysis of Speech Samples (LASS)	75–100 utterances	5–11 years	Engler, Hannah, and Longhurst, 1973
	Assigning Structural Stage (ASS)	At least 50 utterances in at least two contexts	18 months–7 years	Miller, this volume
Semantics	Brown's 14 Grammatical Morphemes	500–700 utterances	2–5 + years	Brown, 1973
	Semantic roles in one-word period	50 + utterances	10–30 months	Chapman, this volume
	Brown's prevalent multi-term semantic relations	50 + utterances	20–48 months	Brown, 1973; Retherford, Schwartz and Chapman, in press
	Semantic relations expressed in conjunctions	50 + utterances	29 months–10 years	Clancy, Jacobsen, and Silva, 1976 (see Table 13)
	Semantic fields: Semantic roles expressed in *Wh*-questions	50 + utterances	18 months–8 years	this volume (see Table 14)
Phonology	Natural process analysis	Representative sample	1–12 years[a]	Ingram, 1976; 1980
	Natural Process Analysis (NPA) Procedure for Phonological Analysis of Continuous Speech Samples	90 words, first occurrence of each	1–12 years[a]	Shriberg and Kwiatkowski, 1980
Communicative Use	Communicative intentions	50 + utterances	10 months +	Chapman, Chapter 4 this volume
	Topic initiation/speaking turn	50 + utterances	10 months +	Bates and Johnston, 1978

[a]Approximate range of use; not specified by author(s)

ing, but this criterion is not consistent for the data from other researchers. The problem of choosing criteria for productivity in child speech is discussed by Ingram (in preparation).

Since some structures develop over a period of time, inconsistent usage across several stages results, and this fact makes specific assignment difficult. For example, the copula appears in Stage II in some form; in Stage III the contractible form was used correctly in 64% of its obligatory contexts, the uncontractible form in 28% by the children studied by de Villiers and de Villiers (1973b). At Stage IV contractible forms were used correctly 67% of the time and uncontractible forms were used correctly 35% of the time. The data document only minimal change in copula development between Stages III and IV. Stage assignments for percent usage similar to Stage III or IV might best be designated as both III–IV. In order to facilitate the use of the charts, however, we have wherever possible adopted the somewhat arbitrary 50% criterion. That is, we call a structure "emerging" when we could adduce that 50% of the subjects in a study used it. Again, the criterion for what constitutes "using" a structure varies from study to study. Also, much of the data in the charts derives from small, longitudinal studies. In those cases it was not possible to use the 50% criterion and we have simply reported the authors' results.

This decision results in somewhat conservative stage assignments. For example, copulas first appear at Stage II, although they don't reach the 90% mastery criterion until Stage V. If copula usage is not 90% correct, then, we can only give the child credit for Stage II development in this aspect of verb phrase elaboration. For this reason, it is especially important to take into account as many aspects of the child's production as possible in the analysis. The 14 morpheme count and the examination of complex sentences can help compensate for the conservative stage assignments in the simple sentence analysis by giving the child credit for higher stage performance in terms of sentence types and mastery of elements that emerge early in simple sentences. There will be variation among these measures, and the overall stage assignment will attempt to take this variation into account.

The focus of our analysis of free-speech sample transcripts has been syntax and semantics. The exclusion of phonology is not intended to minimize its importance. On the contrary, phonological deficits frequently accompany developmental delays in syntax and semantics. There are a number of excellent presentations of phonological analysis procedures already available, however. Examples include distinctive feature analysis (McReynolds and Huston, 1971; Pollack and Rees, 1972), generative phonology (Compton, 1970; Schane, 1973), and natural generative phonology (Ingram, 1976). We have found Ingram's (1981) and Shriberg and Kwiatkowski's (1980) natural process approach particularly helpful in linking developmental phonology with syntax and semantics.

The section that follows provides specific procedures for analyzing syntax and semantics in the framework of Brown's stages, as well as a summary of the developmental data upon which stage assignments can be based. These procedures and data should be considered guides, not recipes, for evaluating language production. Creative applications of the procedures are encouraged. The object of the game is to maximize the child's performance through almost any means, to write it down, and to analyze it in order to create order from randomness. In this way we can arrive at consistent, data-based clinical judgments rather than emotional interpretations.

Analyzing Simple Sentences: Assigning Structural Stage (ASS)

The ASS is a relatively straightforward procedure designed to provide a detailed description of the child's structural development in simple sentences. Its goal is to document the child's stage of development with reference to major grammatical structures. The principle advantage of this kind of procedure is that it allows us to compare the developmental status of each construction produced by the child with the expectations for normal development summarized in a set of charts (see chapter appendix B) that outline the findings of recent research in the acquisition of productive syntax. Assignment of the various structures in the transcript to stages of development allows us to make an overall stage assignment, which is a synthesis of the information on individual structures. This overall stage assignment is then compared to the child's age and MLU in order to decide whether productive syntax appears delayed. The stage designations and the resulting developmental descriptions are specific enough to provide the basis for planning treatment programming when deficits are discovered. The structural development charts can also help establish long-range goals for syntactic therapy.

There is no right way to carry out this procedure. The guidelines presented in this chapter are simply hints that we have found helpful in streamlining the process for efficiency. But there are many ways the ASS can be done and each clinician will find his or her own method of administration. (Table 9, this chapter, and Table 1, Chapter 3, are two sample worksheets for ASS.) The only thing all the procedures have in common is the careful comparison of child utterance to examples in the charts, accurate stage assignments for individual structures, and thoughtful weighing of all the measures taken in arriving at an overall stage assignment. It is important to complete the 14 morpheme analysis before using the structural development charts when determining overall stage assignment.

The 14 Morpheme Analysis A worksheet is necessary for recording the 14 morpheme analysis. The morphemes are placed within stages derived from de Villiers and de Villiers (1973b). Table 8 shows examples of the stage assignments. A completed sample worksheet, analyzing the sample transcript (chapter appendix A) using the 14 morpheme analysis, is shown in Figure 1. Each obligatory context for each morpheme is recorded in the left-hand column. The numbers identify utterances on the transcript. The presence (✓) or absence (–) of a morpheme in the obligatory context is recorded in the right-hand column. The percentage of occurrence for each morpheme is computed by dividing the number of realizations by the number of obligatory contexts.

Note that in counting copulas and auxiliaries, data is provided only for forms of *be*, so only copula and auxiliary *be* forms can be scored. The terms *contractible* and *uncontractible* refer to whether or not the option for contracting the verb exists in Standard English. For example, "I am on my way" or "I'm on my way" are both examples of contractible copulas. Similarly "I'm playing" and "I am playing" are both examples of contractible auxiliaries. Whether or not the verb is actually contracted makes no difference in the stage assignment of contractible forms. Uncontractible copulas and auxiliaries are usually found in sentence-final position and cannot correctly be contracted (Who's there? I *am*. Who's making cookies? I *am*.)

Cazden (1968) described four periods of inflectional development: absence of inflection, occasional production without overgeneralization, increased frequency of occurrence with overgeneralization, and the attainment of 90% correct usage. Brown (1973) adopts the 90% criterion and considers a morpheme "acquired" when it is used correctly in 90% of its obligatory contexts. The highest stage in which the child shows "acquisition" of these morphemes is part of the data for making an overall stage assignment when the analysis is complete. It is important to note that a period of inconsistent usage and overgeneralization precedes mastery in normal children. Inconsistency and overgeneralization in the use of these morphemes should be taken into account during the second part of the ASS, and not simply disregarded as "errors."

The 14 morpheme analysis yields mastery or acquisition data, while most of the structures listed on the structural development charts are placed at their emergence level, or the point at which they first ap-

Table 8. Stage assignments for 14 grammatical morphemes

Stage	Morpheme	Example
II	*-ing*	Me playing.
	plural	That books.
	in	Cookie Monster in there.
III	*on*	Doggie on car.
	possessive	Mommy's shoe.
V	regular past	He walked.
	irregular past	She came.
		We went.
	regular third person singular	It jumps.
		She plays.
	articles *a, the*	That's a puppy.
		Here is the paper.
	contractible copula *be*	Here's my coat.
		Those are my crayons.
V+	contractible auxiliary *be*	They're playing.
		I am coming.
	uncontractible copula *be*	Who's here? I *am*.
	uncontractible auxiliary *be*	Who's playing? I *am*.
	irregular third person singular	She has.
		He does.

Source: de Villiers and de Villiers, 1973b.

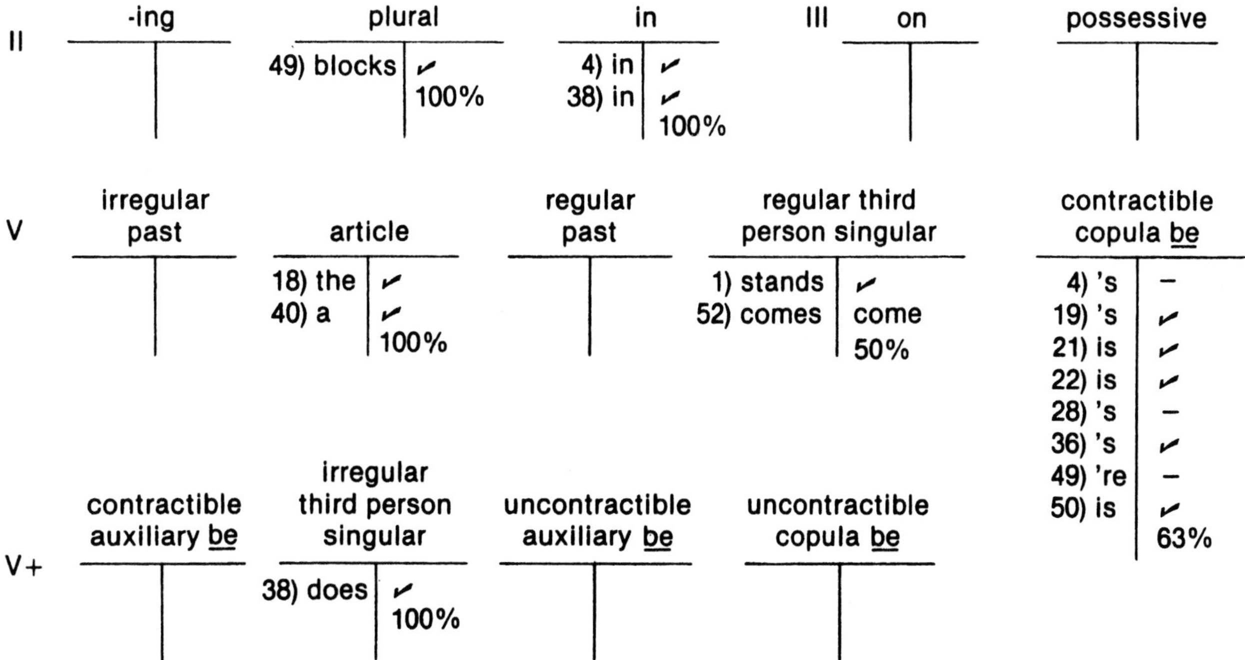

Figure 1. Sample worksheet for recording the analysis of Brown's 14 grammatical morphemes.

pear in child speech but may not be fully mastered. For this reason structures appearing in the charts (chapter appendix B) at the emergence level that also appear in the 14 morpheme count at the mastery level are marked with an asterisk (*). If, after completing the 14 morpheme analysis, it appears that a particular morpheme has been acquired, there is no need to score it at the emergence level when doing the analysis from the charts. Morphemes that do not reach the 90% criterion, however, can be recorded at the emergence level in the second part of the analysis. Overgeneralization can also be noted at that time. For this reason, it is helpful to complete the 14 morpheme analysis before comparing utterances from the transcript to structures in the charts.

Using the Structural Development Charts The first thing to do when assigning structural stage is to read through the charts carefully, examining the structures and example sentences listed there. Becoming familiar with the structures expected at each stage will make the actual analysis much faster and easier.

Next, it is necessary to decide which structural categories are to be analyzed. This is important because it is not always necessary to analyze all possible constructions. Similarly, not all the utterances produced by the child can be analyzed with this procedure. Analysis is restricted to the constructions listed on the charts, which are those for which we have research data available at the time of this writing.

In order to select the structures to be analyzed, several factors must be taken into account. One is MLU, which helps establish which structures we would expect to see. For children with MLUs below 2.5, for example, we would not need to include a complex sentence analysis since very few, if any, complex sentences could be generated in such short utterances. For MLUs over 2.0 we would probably leave out analysis of one-word utterances, since we would have better syntactic data from multi-word sentences.

Another consideration that affects the choice of constructions to be analyzed is the purpose for the analysis. If, for example, we have collateral data that documents a delay, from the DSS perhaps, the ASS might be used to describe specific areas that appear to be problems in the more general analysis, such as questions and negatives. In that case, only these constructions might be investigated. In the sample transcript analysis (chapter appendix A) we have elected to examine the child's use of the basic structural components of simple sentences including noun phrase elaboration, verb phrase elaboration including auxiliary development, negation and questions. Semantic role analysis, using the Retherford, Schwartz, Chapman (in press) scheme is also noted on the sample transcript.

Once the structures to be examined have been identified, it is useful to draw up a worksheet to use in completing the analysis. (See Table 9 for a sample of one of the many forms this worksheet might take.) Structures to be examined in the transcript are placed at their stage assignment (rows) on the worksheet under the structural type they exemplify (columns). We can go through the sample transcript, construction by construction, noting the number of each utterance and placing it beside the structure at the stage it exemplifies. Alternatively, we can go through the transcript, utterance by utterance, noting all the structures that appear within an utterance at one time.

The sample transcript (chapter appendix A) has been analyzed according to the latter procedure and the data transferred to the worksheet (Table 9). Utterance number 1 contains a demonstrative, recorded at Stage III of NP elaboration and a verb inflection scored as one of the 14 morphemes. Utterance numbers 2 and 3 contain no data for the analysis we have set up. Utterance number 4 contains an example of *in*, and a missing copula, scored at Stage I. Utterance number 5 has no scorable data. Utterance number 6 is recorded at Stage III of yes/no question development, since it does not contain a preposed auxiliary, and so on.

Determining Overall Stage Assignment Making an overall stage assignment summarizing performance across constructions may be useful in describing the child's developmental status. However, in making this overall assignment, it is important to bear in mind that the developmental level of individual constructions can vary as much as one, or even, on occasion, two stages on either side of MLU stage assignment or the most frequent level of other structures in the transcript. This kind of variation is expected and occurs frequently in normal children.

Overall stage can be derived in two ways, each summarizing different characteristics. First, the stage of usual performance can be derived by assigning a stage to each construction type—NP elaboration, VP elaboration and so on—according to the frequency with which a stage appears within a type. The stage assignment that appears most frequently for all construction types is selected to summarize the stage of usual performance. Second, the acquisition stage can be derived by summarizing the highest stage assignments for each construction type produced at least once. Alternatively, two stage assignments can be reported, overall usual productive complexity and the complexity level of constructions the child is in the process of acquiring.

When usual performance stage and acquisition stage do not differ, we must ask why. The child's development may have plateaued for a number of reasons, including cognitive or input characteristics. While we have observed children who appear not to be acquiring new structures, we can only speculate as to the significance of the phenomenon relative to prognosis for improvement with intervention. Clearly, we need detailed case studies and controlled intervention research studies to clarify this issue. A lack of consistent performance within structural type, i.e., variation of more than one or two stages that appears completely random without any one stage of performance predominating (which we have rarely observed), is direct evidence for a language disorder rather than a delay in structural acquisition.

The determination of overall stage assignment for the sample transcript is shown below. The child's MLU, 2.50, corresponds to Stage III. Examination of his 14 morpheme analysis (Figure 1) shows him to be 100% correct for Stage II morphemes. There are no instances of Stage III, and inconsistent use of regular third person singular and contractible copulas at Stage V. Use of articles is 100%, and one instance of irregular third person singular is correct. It is important not to overcredit this one instance of correct performance since we know children often master individual irregular forms early, then lose them when they learn a productive rule for generating the form. Irregular forms are then reacquired as exceptions to the rule at a later stage. Since there are no other instances of irregular third person forms, we have no way of deciding whether this is an early memorized form or an instance of an exception to a productive rule. For this reason, we could conclude that the child is acquiring Stage V morphemes because he is showing 50%-60% correct performance on verb forms of Stage V and 100% on articles.

Examining his performance on the simple sentence analysis from the worksheet (Table 9) shows that most of his structures are at Stage III or below, although Stage IV questions do appear. We would credit the child with a usual level of performance at Stage III, with acquisition proceeding into Stage IV for questions and Stage V for grammatical morphemes. This performance seems perfectly consistent with what we would expect for an MLU of 2.50. But when we refer to the child's chronological age we see that he is 6;8, much older than the predicted age for an MLU in Stage III. Because his production is so typical of a Stage III child despite his advanced age, we can be confident in calling him significantly delayed, but not deviant, in language.

Although it is true that we could have made the same diagnosis simply on the basis of this child's MLU, it is important to notice what *else* we have

Table 9. ASS Summary Worksheet

Name: ______ MLU: 2.50 Age: 6–8 Number of Utterances: 52 Date: ______

Stage	Noun phrase elaboration	Verb phrase elaboration	Negatives	Questions
I	NP→(M) + N alone only:	Unmarked verb: 44, 52 Absent aux: Absent copula: 4, 28, 49	{no / not} + {(NP) / (VP)}	Wh: routines: *what, what do, where*
II	(M) + N in object position: 28	Main verb marked: 1, 38 *-ing* without *be:* Catenative alone: Copula appears: 19, 21, 22, 36, 50	*Neg→no, not, can't, don't:*	Wh: novel:
III	NP→ {demonstrative / article} + (M) + N Demonstratives: 1, 24, 25, 38, 45 *a, the* appear: Quantifiers: 44 Possessives: Adjectives: 40	Pres. aux: *can, will, be:* Overgen'l of *-ed:*	*won't:*	Wh: aux appears without inversion: *why, who, how:* Yes/no: rising intonation: 6, 8, 9, 14, 16, 18, 24, 26, 27, 51
IV	NP→ {demo / art. / (M) / poss} + adj. + N:	Main V and aux doubly Marked for past in neg: Past modals: Catenative + NP: *Be + -ing:*	Neg→pres. *be, can, will, do, did, does:*	Wh: *do* appears: aux: inverted: 19, 21, 22, 36, 50 *when:* Yes/no: aux inverted: *Do* appears: 38
V		V + : Past *be:* *Have + en:*	Neg→past *be,* past modals:	

learned from the ASS. First, all the analysis supports the conclusion that the child is structurally delayed and not just uncommunicative. His sentence structures are consistently simple with relatively few falling above the level predicted by MLU. Second, we see some strengths: The child can produce well-formed questions. We might decide in planning therapy that questions would be an appropriate context in which to expand the child's use of auxiliary forms and verb inflections. Using a modeling approach, we might take the question forms he does have ("What's that?" "Does it. . .?") and model the same forms with different verbs ("What are those?") or different question words ("Where is that?") and so on. The examination of ASS data gives us more than just a stage assignment. It allows us to interpret the child's performance and to infer strengths and weakness that will be relevant in prescribing a syntactic therapy program.

Analyzing Complex Sentence Development *by Rhea Paul*

The complex sentence development charts (chapter appendix C, pages 67–71), which outline some milestones in development of complex sentence production, are based on an analysis of transcripts of the speech of 59 children between the ages of 2;5 and 6;11 who are engaged in 15-minute free-play sessions with their mothers. The mother-child sessions were videotaped and transcribed by Dr. Susan Wanska, who also calculated MLU for both the children and their mothers. Dr. Wanska was kind enough to make her transcripts and MLU calculations available for the analysis that led to the development of these charts.

In order to perform the analysis, the children were placed in five groups according to their MLU using 0.5 morpheme intervals: 3.00–3.50 (N=16), 3.51–4.00 (N=15), 4.01–4.50 (N=13), 4.51–5.00 (N=8), and 5.01–up (N=7). Each transcript was examined for the appearance of various forms of embedding, conjoining, and individual conjunctions. The proportion of subjects within each MLU grouping that used each form at least once was then calculated. The charts indicate the first MLU stage in which at least 50% of the children in a group used a structure. In some cases, the same structure reached usage by 90% of the subjects in a higher group. When this occurred, it is also shown on the charts. This procedure follows that used by Chapman (in preparation) to arrive at stage placements for simple sentence constructions.

Regression analyses performed on the data show MLU to be a better predictor of use of most types of complex sentences than either age or cognitive level. This result supports the conclusion that an increase in the use of different types of complex sentences is related to increases in MLU. Three types of embeddings were too infrequent to show a significant relation to MLU. These clause types are included in the charts but are marked with a dagger (†) indicating that although their use also increased with MLU, the increase was not statistically significant.

Two main classes of complex sentences are dealt with in the charts. Both types are mainly characterized by the fact that they contain more than one main verb. The first class consists of conjoined sentences. These are made up of two or more full sentences connected within one utterance, usually by a conjunction such as *and, but, so, before,* or *after.* In the early stages, however, some children may connect two sentences in an utterance without using any conjunction at all simply by juxtaposing the clauses without an intonation boundary. These sentences are also counted as conjoined. The charts show that children first join only two sentences or independent clauses. At a later stage, they can combine the two types of complex sentences, embedded and conjoined, within one utterance.

The second type of complex sentence, the embedded, contains a clause, that is, a sentence-like segment that contains a main verb, within a larger sentence. In embedded sentences, the clause is not independent, but serves as a constituent part of the main, or matrix, sentence. The clause may act as the subject, for example, as in "*What I'm doing* is writing." Often it functions as a direct object, as in "You can see *what I'm doing.*" The following types of embedding were found to reach the criterion of at least one use by over 50% of the subjects in the MLU grouping listed as the stage of emergence for that type on the charts:

---

let's, let me:

These clause introducers appear to operate somewhat as unanalyzed catenatives do, and are therefore considered as forms rather than structures.

Example: *Let's* get in.
Let me see.

Simple infinitive clauses with equivalent subjects:

These include clauses marked by *to* in which the subject of the clause is the same as that of the main sentence. The subject of the clause does not usually appear, because it would be redundant. (This category does *not* include the catenative, or the semi-auxiliary forms *gonna, gotta, wanna, hafta,* or *s'posedta,* which appear to function as unanalyzed wholes and are considered in the simple sentence analysis.)

Examples: He has *to move.*
I need new glasses *to read.*
I'll get the rocking chair for me *to sit on.*
I like *to hear that.*
It gots *to go down here.*

Full propositional complements:
These clauses contain a complete surface sentence. They usually follow a verb such as *know, wonder, guess, think, pretend, forget, say, mean, tell, remember,* or *wish.* The clause may or may not begin with *that,* but does not begin with a Wh-word.

Examples: I think *it is right.*
She said *that I can do it.*
Pretend *that's grass.*
I forgot *you need a truck.*

Simple non-infinitive Wh-clauses:
These clauses begin with a Wh-word such as *when, what, where, why, how, if,* or *like.* They do not contain the infinitive marker *to.*

Examples: See *if it can go on this track.*
He doesn't know *where he's going.*
Do it *like I do it.*
You know *what this is?*
That's *how you do it.*

†Infinitive clauses with different subjects:
The subject of the infinitive clause is not the same as that of the main sentence. The subject of the clause usually does appear.

Examples: How do you get *this to stay on?*
That's for *you to do.*
You want *me to wind it up?*
I got some more tea for *her to drink.*

Relative clauses:
These modify nouns. They can be marked by *which, who, that,* or *what* in child speech, but often do not contain any relative pronoun at all.

Examples: Could we take the pictures home *that we drew?*
Look at the big bubble *I made.*
They're boys *what you know.*

†Gerund clauses:
These contain *-ing* verbs. The *-ing* form must be part of a noun clause. The *-ing* adjectives, as in *Let's play with the stacking cups,* are not considered instances of gerund clauses for the purpose of this analysis.

Examples: I can almost climb up that high one without *climbing on the foot.*
I was trying to get this stuff off by *washing my hands.*
Look at *him moving around.*

Unmarked infinitive clauses:
These do not contain *to* in the surface sentence and are usually headed by *make, help, watch,* or *let.*

Examples: I'll make *the ball stay on that chair.*
You help *us do this.*
I'll let *you try.*
Watch *me run the train.*

†Wh-infinitive clauses:
These are marked by both a Wh-word and *to.*

Examples: Do you know *how to play it now?*
Tell me *when to start.*
I'll show *you what to do.*

Double embeddings:
An embedded clause is contained within another embedded clause, which is in turn embedded in a matrix sentence. One of these clauses may include a catenative.

Examples: I think *I know what this is.*
I'm gonna *let it go now.*
You hafta *try to find one like this.*

Each of the five MLU stages in chapter appendix C contains five sections. Section 1 shows the percentage of true complex sentences a speech sample at that stage will probably contain. The percentage of true complex sentences is calculated by dividing the number of complex sentences in the sample—*excluding* those that contain only the catenative forms *gonna, gotta, wanna, hafta, s'posedta, let's* or *let me*—by the total number of utterances. This percentage does not always change with every MLU increment, and cannot be used alone to determine stage assignment. It must be considered in conjunction with the other indices.

Section 2 shows the forms of embedding that reach criterion for each stage. The forms that are marked with an asterisk (*) at the 50% level will appear again at a later stage, indicating they are used by 90% of the subjects in a higher MLU group. Not every structure reaches 90% usage, however.

Section 3 deals with the appearance of conjoined sentences. It also shows when sentences that contain both conjoined and embedded clauses within one utterance reach criterion. Examples of such sentences are: "I'm gonna erase it *'cause* I don't want *you to have a D for a head*" and "She had *to take him* 'cause he was a little bit shy."

Section 4 shows when specific conjunctions reach either the 50% or 90% criterion in the sample. Section 5 deals with the average number of different conjunctions that appear in the 15-minute samples. These are conjunction types, not tokens. If *and* appears six times in a sample, for instance, it is only counted once. There is quite a bit of variability among children within an MLU grouping on both these conjunction measures. Again, they should not be used alone to determine stage assignment, but only as a part of the overall picture of the child's language production.

The complex sentence analysis can be done along with the simple sentence procedure (ASS) outlined in chapter appendix B, or it can be done separately. For children with MLUs above 4.5, the simple sentence analysis will probably only provide a baseline level, and the analysis of the complex sentence will be the major factor in overall stage placement in most cases. For children with MLUs between 3.0 and 4.5, complex sentence analysis will most likely serve to supplement the simple sentence procedure. It is possible that even children with MLUs below 4.5 will show more evidence of linguistic growth in their complex sentence use than they do in simple sentences. When this happens it is up to the clinician to decide on which index—complex or simple sentences—to place the greater weight. A suggested procedure for using the complex sentence development charts to augment the analysis of the speech samples is shown below. Certainly other procedures are possible, and each clinician using the charts will develop the method he or she finds most efficient. The procedure suggested here allows most of the complex sentence analysis to be done concurrently with that of simple sentences. The step-by-step guidelines are not meant to imply that no other means of proceeding is valid. They are offered only as a way of familiarizing clinicians with material that may be new to them. (A sample worksheet for this concurrent analysis is provided in Table 10. To use it, one simply goes through the transcript, sentence by sentence, assigning both simple and complex utterances to the stage shown in the charts.)

Procedure for Using the Complex Sentence Development Charts

Step 1: *Decide whether to use the 50% or 90% criterion in assigning structures in the script to stages.* The 50% criterion is perhaps more convenient, since it is present for every item that appears on the charts. Some structures never reach the 90% level. However, the 50% level is more conservative. For any structure at the 50% level, obviously, half of the children in that MLU group *never* use it. The 90% criterion gives the child more of the benefit of the doubt, in that it gives him credit for a higher stage. The 90% level is perhaps the measure of choice when the clinician is deciding whether or not a child has a problem and does not want to risk calling him delayed when he may only be on the slow side of normal.

Step 2: *Identify each complex sentence in the transcript as you go through the sample assigning the simple sentences to stages.* Mark the true complex sentences so they can be counted later. Identify the form of each embedded or conjoined sentence. Then find the stage on the charts at which that form reaches the chosen criterion (50% or 90%). If a worksheet (similar to Table 10) is used, note the utterance's number beside the corresponding form on the worksheet. When the analysis is completed, the worksheet can be scanned to determine the stage in which the greatest number of utterances fall in order to make a stage assignment.

Step 3: *Identify each conjunction used in the sample.* Find the stage at which each one reaches criterion on the charts. Some conjunctions in your sample may not appear on the charts because they did not reach criterion in the data base. Mark the conjunctions that do appear on the charts in the appropriate stage on the worksheet.

Step 4: *Count the number of different conjunctions in the sample.* Count only the first appearance of each conjunction. Place the total number at the stage to which it corresponds on the charts. (Note that there is quite a bit of variability within each MLU group on the two conjunction measures.)

Step 5: *Calculate the percentage of true complex sentences (exclude sentences containing only* gonna, gotta, wanna, hafta, spozta, let's, *and* let me). Find the

Table 10. ASS / Complex Sentence Summary Worksheet

Name: ______ MLU: 3.20 Age: 41 months Number of Utterances: 136 Date: ______

Stage	Verb phrase elaboration	Negatives	Questions	Complex sentences
I	Unmarked V: 39 Absent aux: Absent copula:	no + NP not + VP	Wh: routines: *what, what do, where:*	Criterion: 50% 90%
II	Main V marked: *-ing* without *be:* Catenative alone: Copula appears: 53, 57	Neg→*no, not, can't, don't:* 39, 98	Wh: novel: 89	
III	Aux: present *Can:* 38, 99 *Will:* 56, 117 *Be:* 122, 133 Overgen'l *ed:* 5, 18	Neg→*won't:*	Wh: aux, without inversions: 14 *why, who, how:* Y/n: rising intonation: 118	
Early IV	Past modals: 5 *Be + -ing:* 94 Catenative + NP: 9, 24, 42, 53, 55, 56, 92	Neg→ pres. *be, can, will, do, did, does:*	Wh: *do* appears: Aux inverted: 19 *When:* Y/n: *do* appears: Aux inverted:	1. 1–10%: 2. Simple inf: 2, 3, 67 full: 4 *let's, let me:* Wh: 9 3. 2 conjoined: 5 4. *and:* 5. 0–4:
Late IV Early V		Neg→past *be,* past modal:		1. 1–10%: 2. Double embedding: 3. Conjoin and embed in one s: 4. — 5. 1–5:
Late V				1. 10–20%: 2. Inf. dif. subj. relatives 3. — 4. *if* 5. 2–6:
V+	past *be:* *Have + -en:*			1. 10–20%: 2. Gerunds: Wh-inf: 10 unmarked inf: 1 3. — 4. *because:* 5 5. 2–6:
V++				1. Over 20%: 2. — 3. — 4. When: *so:* 5. 6–8:

stage to which this percentage corresponds. (Note that there is some overlap.)

Step 6: Assign an overall stage to the transcript by combining information from MLU, simple and complex sentence analyses, and 14 morpheme analysis. Use either the usual performance criterion (the most frequent stage) or the acquisition criterion (the highest stage that appears), depending on the purpose of the analysis. If the acquisition criterion is used, be wary of relying on the two conjunction indices (Sections 4 and 5 on the charts) alone, because there is so much within-group variation on these two measures. If either of them falls above all the other indices, it is probably wise to choose the next highest stage as the level of emerging structures.

Sample Analysis

A 41-month-old child was the subject of the complex sentence analysis. (See Table 10 for a sample worksheet.) Her MLU was 3.20 and her speech sample contained 136 utterances. The analysis of her simple sentences, which also appears in the worksheet, places her at Stage III to Early Stage IV. A transcript of only her true complex sentences, upon which the complex sentence stage assignment of her speech sample is determined, is shown below.

Transcript of True Complex Sentences

1. Let you try.
2. She wants to get out.
3. She wants to have call by baby.
4. The doctor says that baby's crying.
5. Don't push that button-like thing 'cause that would. . . it operated.
6. I got go home now.
7. It gots to go down here.
8. It go fall down boom.
9. I don't know what it is.
10. You know how to teach this?

Analysis

Structure	Stage Assignment: (50% level)
1. Percentage of true complex sentences:	
10/136 = 7%	IV–V
2. Forms of embedding:	
#1-unmarked infinitive clause	V+
#2-simple infinitive (also #3, 6, 7, 8)	IV
#4-full propositional clause	IV
#9-simple Wh-clause	IV
#10-Wh-infinitive clause	V+
3. Forms of conjoining:	
two clauses only (#5)	IV
4. Conjunctions used:	
because	V+
5. Number of different conjunctions:	
1	IV–V

Using the usual performance criterion for overall stage assignment, in combination with this child's MLU and her stage placement for simple sentences, this child would be assigned to Stage IV. In order to decide whether this child has a language problem we refer to her chronological age, 41 months. Since this age falls within one standard deviation from the mean age predicted by her MLU ($\overline{X}$=34–37 months, ±1 SD=31–41 months), since she is showing the emergence of some higher level forms (the conjunction *because*, unmarked infinitives, and Wh-infinitives), and since the conservative 50% criterion was used for assigning stages, one can feel confident in concluding that her language is developing at a rate that is within normal range.

SEMANTIC ANALYSES

As children grow older, they both expand and change the aspects of a situation that they choose to talk about. At the present time we have no single system that clearly reflects these changes. We have a patchwork of categories, some helpful for one kind of development and some for another.

In exploring the growth and change in meanings children express, it is important to be clear about the distinctions among semantics and the other developing systems with which it interacts. One such distinction is between the underlying concepts the child is acquiring as he or she grows (cognition) and the means for expressing these concepts in words (semantics). In this volume, we are primarily concerned with language assessment, and not the evaluation of intellectual development, which will be explored in a later volume in this series. For the present purposes, we will want to evaluate only the child's expression of meanings through language. Cognitive assessment is often useful in setting goals for language therapy, particularly in mentally retarded populations, since it helps us establish very general expectations for language performance. But in analyzing the semantic component of a child's language system we must know more than what meanings cognitive level would predict to be expressed. We must find out what the child actually can and does talk about.

Semantics is a very elusive subject because it overlaps so generously with both syntax and pragmatics. For example, many of the early semantic roles that have been studied in child language—agent, action, object, and so on—are both semantic and syntactic in that they not only characterize the meaning of the words that fill the slots, they represent something about their grammatical function as well. Agents are almost always subjects of sentences. And the consistent word order used in expressing these roles also reflects that the child knows more than meaning categories. The child knows these categories must be combined in a certain (grammatical) structure, or sequence, in order to express the desired meaning. Bloom and Lahey (1978) refer to these early semantic role combinations as "semantic-syntactic" relations. When we evaluate semantic performance in children we want to try to tease out the specifically semantic component of the grammar to as great an extent as possible.

Similarly, semantics and pragmatics overlap in that it is often very difficult to separate the meaning of a sentence from its use. Indirect requests, such as "Can you pass the salt?," are a classic example of this problem, since their literal meaning ("Are you able to pass the salt?") is not what the speaker intends the listener to understand by the utterance. In analyzing the semantic component of a child's production it is important to keep these problems in mind.

This section can only present a very limited introduction to the task of exploring a child's use of semantic knowledge. Many semantic taxonomies have been presented in the developmental literature, but little work has been done in applying these taxonomies to clinical populations as diagnostic tools. Nor is there at the time of this writing a clear developmental sequence for the acquisition of semantic expression beyond the period of Brown's Stages I or II. For these reasons we are unable to present clinic-tested semantic analysis procedures. All we can do is provide a framework for thinking about semantic development and refer the reader to some normative studies that may prove useful in setting up experimental analysis protocols.

De Villiers and de Villiers (1978) proposed a distinction between referential meaning and relational meaning in discussing semantic development. Referential meaning is that which concerns the primarily one-to-one link between words and the objects or concepts they stand for. Relational meaning has to do with the connections among concepts, words, and sentences.

Referential Meaning

For our purposes, referential meaning is primarily explored through analysis of the child's use of individual words. Two analyses might be used here, the type-token ratio, and semantic field analysis. The type-token ratio indexes lexical diversity. Templin (1957) presents a procedure for calculating vocabulary usage based on the *number of different words* produced in a 50-utterance sample and the *total number of words* produced in such a sample (see Table 11). The relationship between these two measures is calculated by dividing the total number of words used into the total number of different words. The resulting number is called a type (number of different word types used)-token (number of total word tokens used) ratio (TTR). Templin reports that for the 480 children she studied, ratios of approximately 1:2 (or a TTR of 0.50) occurred consistently across all age groups, sex groups, and socioeconomic status (SES). The consistency of this measure makes it enormously valuable as a clinical tool. For example, if a normal hearing child's TTR is significantly below 0.50 we can be reasonably certain the sparseness of vocabulary use is *not* an artifact of SES but is probably indicative of a language-specific deficiency.

Table 11. Calculating vocabulary diversity using type-token ratio. N = 480

Age	Different words Mean	Different words SD	Total words Mean	Total words SD	Type-token ratio (Different words ÷ total words)
3.0	92.5	26.1	204.9	61.3	0.45
3.5	104.8	20.4	232.9	50.8	0.45
4.0	120.4	27.6	268.8	72.6	0.45
4.5	127.0	23.9	270.7	65.3	0.47
5.0	132.4	27.2	286.2	75.5	0.46
6.0	147.0	27.6	328.0	65.9	0.45
7.0	157.7	27.2	363.1	51.3	0.43
8.0	166.5	29.5	378.8	80.9	0.44

From: Mildred C. Templin, *Certain Language Skills in Children.* Copyright ©1957 by the University of Minnesota. University of Minnesota Press, Minneapolis.

Type-token ratios are easy to compute from transcripts and provide a handy means of quantifying vocabulary. It is important to remember that TTRs can only be compared to Templin's data for children 3 through 8 years of age.

The following procedures for computing type-token ratios (Templin, 1957) should be followed as closely as possible to ensure that the data collected are comparable to Templin's.

I. Utterance sample (Templin, 1957, p. 15) Templin employed McCarthy's (1930) procedures in collecting speech samples. She used picture books and toys as stimulus materials in an adult-child interaction context. Fifty consecutive utterances were recorded (handwritten, on-line) after the child was comfortable and rapport had been established. Utterance boundaries were determined by a "natural break in the verbalization of the child."

II. Rules for counting number of words (Templin, 1957, p. 160)
   A. Contractions of subject and predicate like *it's* and *we're* are counted as two words.
   B. Contractions of the verb and the negative such as *can't* are counted as one word.
   C. Each part of a verbal combination is counted as a separate word: Thus "have been playing" is counted as three words.
   D. Hyphenated and compound nouns are one word.
   E. Expressions that function as a unit in the child's understanding are counted as one word. Thus *oh boy, all right,* etc., are counted as one word, while *Christmas tree* is counted as two words.
   F. Articles *the, a, an* count as one word.
   G. Bound morphemes and noun and verb inflections are not counted as separate words.

III. Computing TTRs
   A. Identify 50 consecutive utterances from the transcript, preferably the middle 50.
   B. Count total number of words expressed employing the rules in II above.
   C. Count total number of different words expressed.
   D. Divide total number of different words by total number of words expressed. The result is the TTR.

Semantic field analysis provides another way of looking at the range of the child's vocabulary. Here we have no standardized procedure, but have to create a set of meaning categories for the words that appear in the transcript. We might use such categories as animals, people, vehicles, and buildings for nouns. Movement, existence, desire, etc., might categorize verbs. Modifiers such as adjectives and adverbs may be particularly enlightening in establishing the complexity of the ideas the child expresses. We would expect the expression of notions of duration (long, short), temporal sequence (first, last), manner (hard, loud), and distance (far, near) to be associated with relatively later cognitive development, certainly later than the period of Stage I–II semantic role combinations. If these notions are encoded by children with low levels of structural development, we could predict a discrepancy between their cognitive and linguistic performance. More generally, semantic field analysis gives us another way of talking about the diversity and complexity of the child's vocabulary in terms both of number of meaning categories and different words within categories.

Another aspect of referential meaning that can be explored is the expression of advanced notions of space and time. These notions are somewhat difficult to specify since it is often hard to identify them reliably in particular words or constructions.

The utterance "The car hit the bus" expresses an action that is ongoing or just complete if produced in the clinic room to describe a play event. The same utterance produced in response to questions may give evidence of comprehension of notions of time and space. For example, if the adult asks "What happened yesterday?" and the child responds, "The car hit the bus," he or she indicates that the request (what significant event happened on the preceding day) was understood. This request for information requires the understanding of the lexical time marker *yesterday* and the ability to recall and report the event referred to. The request "What happened at Grandma's?" requires the child to understand that Grandma resides in a place other than the child's home, a generally spatial notion, to determine the reference to past time, and to recall the significant event.

The development of the ability to think and talk about events removed from the present is a complex sequence and has not been explored in detail developmentally. There is some evidence suggesting that children express spatial notions before temporal notions, noting immediate, present events before past events before future events. Specific lexical quantification of time—seconds, minutes, hours, days, weeks, months—occurs quite late in the preoperational or the early concrete operational period. The prepositional phrase, first used in English to express spatial notions, is later used to express time notions: "The car hit the bus on the bridge", "The car hit the bus on April 27th."

While temporal and spatial notions are difficult to quantify and interpret, they are important indicators of possible discrepancies between notions the child can conceive of and those the child can talk about. We would not expect a child whose productions are typical of Stage I syntax to express notions transcending the here-and-now. A child at MLU 1.71 produced the following series of one- and two-word utterances: *All done. Go home. Eat. TV.* This string could be interpreted in context to express that the child is finished with the present activity, wants to change locations, and in the new location wants to eat and then watch TV. The temporal and spatial notions expressed are far more advanced than the form used to express them. Stage I children generally talk about present, immediate events and produce successive single-word utterances usually marking characteristics of a single event. For example, *Man. Coat. Hat.;* meaning the man has a coat and a hat on. (The single-word period of development is described in detail in chapter appendix B.) This example comes from the transcript of a 4-year-old deaf child with an MLU of 1.71. While we cannot document the exact level of semantic development in this child, the expression of advanced semantic notions relative to syntactic form is significant for program planning. Clearly, programming should focus on developing appropriate grammatical structures to express the semantic notions within the child's repertoire.

In trying to investigate the child's knowledge of temporal and spatial relations in cases where we might suspect a discrepancy between grammatical and conceptual abilities, as with deaf children, the clinician can increase the chances of finding such notions encoded in a speech sample by introducing topics about absent objects and events. The judicious use of questions that request such information can be helpful if care is taken not to overload the interaction with adult requests for information.

Relational Meaning

In thinking about the semantics of relational meaning, we can conceive of at least three levels of analysis: intrasentence relations, intersentence relations, and contextual, or nonlinguistic, relations. At the intrasentence level, the most extensively studied aspect of semantic development is the semantic roles coded in children's early two- and three-word combinations (Brown, 1970, 1973; Schlesinger, 1971; Bloom, 1973; Greenfield and Smith, 1976; Retherford, Schwartz, and Chapman, in press). Although there are many relations children could talk about in 2–3 word sentences, it appears that they actually produce a rather restricted number. Brown (1973) presents a set of prevalent relations to look for in the speech of children in Stages I–II. The scheme used by Retherford, Schwartz, and Chapman (definitions of semantic categories are listed in Table 12) has been used to code the relations in the sample transcript, chapter appendix A. Careful consideration should be given to undertaking the semantic role analysis for children above Stage II because we have no developmental data to indicate what kinds of changes in roles encoded we should expect to see in normal children. If we encountered children with longer utterances still only coding the early relations found in Stage I–II and no others, we might suspect either a cognitive or cognitive/semantic disability, but we could not make a definitive diagnosis because there are no data on the normal acquisition of semantic roles to assure us that our suspicion is correct. If, on the other hand, a Stage I–II child is producing two- to three-word utterances but coding only a few of the relations the literature reports to be predominant, the expression of a broader subset of the early roles might be chosen as a target for therapy. And if children with MLUs in the Stage I–II range can be shown to be talking about manner, duration, frequency, causality, temporality, and other relations missing from the early lists we would want to explore their cognitive development to validate the hunch that the child's understanding of the world is more complex than his or her language structures indicate. This finding would also have important implications for programming, since our goal might then be to teach the child some more conventional means for expressing the ideas he or she already has in mind.

Table 12. Definitions of the 21 semantic categories (Retherford, Schwartz, and Chapman, In press)

Action[a] A perceivable movement or activity engaged in by an agent (animate or inanimate).

Entity (One-term utterances only) Any labeling of the present person or object regardless of the occurrence or nature or action being performed on or by it.

Entity (Multi-term utterances only) The use of an appropriate label for a person or object in the absence of any action on it (with the exception of showing, pointing, touching, or grasping); or someone or something which caused or was the stimulus to the internal state specified by a state verb or any object or person which was modified by a possessive form. (**Entity** was used to code a possession if it met either of the preceding criteria).

Locative The place where an object or action was located or toward which it moved.

Negation[b] The impression of any of the following meanings with regard to someone or something, or an action or state: non-existence, rejection, cessation, denial, disappearance.

Agent The performer (animate or inanimate) of an action. Body parts and vehicles, when used in conjunction with action verbs, were coded **Agent.**

Object A person or thing (marked by the use of a noun or pronoun) that received the force of an action.

Demonstrative The use of demonstrative pronouns or adjectives, *this, that, these, those,* and the words *there, right there, here, see,* when stated for the purpose of pointing out a particular referent.

Recurrence A request for or comment on an additional instance or amount; the resumption of an event; or the reappearance of a person or object.

Attribute An adjectival description of the size, shape, or quality of an object or person; also, noun adjuncts which modified nouns for a similar purpose (e.g., *gingerbread* man).

Possessor A person or thing (marked by the use of a proper noun or pronoun) that an object was associated with or to which it belonged, at least temporarily.

Adverbial[c] Included in this category were the two subcategories of action/attribute and state/attribute.

- **Action/Attribute** A modifier of an action indicating time, manner, duration, distance, or frequency. (Direction or place of action was separately coded as **Locative, Repetition** and **Recurrence**).
- State/Attribute A modifier indicating time, manner, quality, or intensity of a state.

Quantifier A modifier which indicated amount or number of a person or object. Prearticles and indefinite pronouns such as *a piece of, lots of, any, every,* and *each* were included.

State A passive condition experienced by a person or object. This category implies involuntary behavior on the part of the **Experiencer,** in contrast to voluntary action performed by an **Agent.**

Experiencer Someone or something that underwent a given experience or mental state. Body parts, when used in conjunction with state verbs, were coded **Experiencer.**

Recipient One who received or was named as the recipient of an *object* (person or thing) from another.

Beneficiary One who benefitted from or was named as the beneficiary of a specified action.

Name The labeling or request for naming of a person or thing using the utterance forms: *my* (*his, your,* etc.) *name is* _______ or *what's* _______ *name?*

Created Object Something created by a specific activity, for example a *song* by singing, a *house* by building, a *picture* by drawing.

Comitative One who accompanied or participated with an agent in carrying out a specified activity.

Instrument Something which an **Agent** used to carry out or complete a specified action.

These categories are used in the sample transcript, chapter appendix A.

[a]Other systems (Chafe, 1970) distinguish action, process, change of state and state categories.

[b]Negation collapsed the following semantic categories: rejection, disappearance, cessation, non-existence, and denial.

[c]This too is a collapse of semantic categories. In addition to the categories coded separately (location, place and direction, recurrence) a semantic breakdown would include: time, distance, duration, frequency, intensity, and manner.

More complex semantic relations also expressed at the intrasentence level are those coded by conjunctions joining two propositions within one utterance. Brown (1973) reports that these conjoined sentences appear first in Stage IV. Initially children join two ideas simply by juxtaposing them, without using any conjunction. In these early conjoinings the same semantic relations are expressed as those coded later by surface conjunctions. But the listener must infer the particular relation meant, since it is not marked overtly.

Clancy, Jacobsen, and Silva (1976) studied children from 1;2 to 4;8 years of age who were acquiring four different languages and found a consistent order of emergence of semantic relations coded in early conjoined sentences despite differences in the formal means of expression in the languages examined. This order of acquisition is shown in Table 13. In a longitudinal study of four children learning English, Hood, Lahey, Lifter, and Bloom (1978) reported a similar order where coding categories were similar, although Hood et al. only examined sentences where connectives were marked on the surface.

While the data in the acquisition of semantic relationships expressed by conjunctions is sparse, it is presented here to point out some of the ways form and meaning interact. Children initially conjoin sen-

Table 13. Semantic relationships expressed in early conjoined sentences

Semantic relation	Form	Age first expressed		Example
Coordination	No surface marker	2;0[a]	2;3[b]	My paper. . . pencil
Sequence	No surface marker	2;0	2;4	Bye-bye, daddy, Karen, Ginger
Antithesis	No surface marker	2;0	2;9	No eat. . . I play
Causality[c] (Logical)	No surface marker	2;0	2;10	I can't do it. I not big enough.
Reasons (Psychological causality)	Because		2;11	You're like that, because you didn't know me.
Temporal relations	Then			Now I go eat. . . Then I play again.
	When	2;8	3;2	When he goes to sleep he reads.
Conditionality	While	3;4	3;3	I wear this while walking.
Temporal sequence	After		3;5	Can I make him a tree, after I finish this?
			4;0	You better move your legs, before I run over your legs.

[a]English cross-sectional data N = 13 (Clancy, Jacobsen, and Silva, 1976)
[b]English longitudinal data N = 1 (Clancy et al., 1976)
[c]For a detailed account of the development of early expressions of causality see: Hood, and Bloom, 1979.

tences by simple juxtaposition without a surface conjunction and express the same semantic relationships that later appear with surface markers.

An examination of semantic relations coded in conjoined sentences can accompany the complex sentence analysis. After the conjoined sentences in the transcript have been identified, the sentences can be analyzed for semantic relations, coded, and these relations compared to the data in Table 13. Although we would not expect to see all possible relations talked about in a 15-minute sample, looking at the range will give some idea of the diversity of relational concepts the child has in mind. We can also explore whether the children are using conjunctions to mark these relations, which is a more advanced stage than using simple juxtaposition, and whether the conjunctions used are the correct ones to mark the intended meaning. The number of different conjunctions used and stage assignments for individual conjunction types derived from the complex sentence analysis will also give some idea of the level of semantic diversity and complexity of which the child is capable.

One last aspect of intrasentence relations a semantic analysis might explore is found in children's requests. Request forms offer a distinct group of utterances expressed with the intention of bringing about a desired state of affairs, or eliciting specific information. The meanings expressed in these utterances are of considerable value in understanding the child's desires to modify the environment, needs requiring satisfaction, and information requested. The frequency, type, and content of requests provide a potential index of the child's curiosity about his or her environment and the degree of control exercised in conversation. This information is the domain of the pragmatic analysis.

The specific content of requests can also provide a general index of semantic development if motivation and conversational control characteristics are kept in mind. Frequency of requests has little to do with semantic content, but the semantic content of requests that do occur can provide another index of semantic diversity and complexity.

Requests can be divided into two general types. Requests for action are usually expressed in imperative form. Requests for information are usually questions. Little developmental data exists on requests for action except that they precede requests for information before and including Stage I, 10–18 months (Bates, 1976). Requests for action do not require words and can be identified reliably through communicative gestures, which may or may not include accompanying vocalizations. Again, this analysis would more properly be considered pragmatic.

Requests for information are usually expressed directly with Wh-question forms. Specific Wh-words indicate the kind of information requested. Table 14 lists question forms and Wh-words with the specific semantic notions requested by each where the data are available. Question-form development from Stage I through Stage V reflects change in the specific information requested, with objects and actions preceding cause and time.

Analysis of specific Wh-words expressed in questions will provide a description of the variety of information requested. Care should be taken not to overinterpret the absence of specific question forms. Questions occur relatively infrequently in children's conversations with adults. Introducing topics about

Table 14. Semantic information requested by question forms

Question type	Developmental stage	Semantic information requested	Predicted age
Yes/No What What do Where (Place) Where (Direction)	Stage I and II	Confirmation Object Action Location Location	19-28 months ± 1 SD = 16-34 months
Whose Who Why How	Stage III infrequently produced	Possessor Person Cause or reason Manner, instrument	31-34 months ± 1 SD = 24-41 months
When	Early Stage IV	Time	35-42 months ± 1 SD = 28-45 months
How many How much How long How far How often How long	No Data Might expect them to appear at the same time as manner adverbials. Expressing the same semantic notions. *How long* may be specific to the acquisition of specific time units: days, weeks, hours, minutes, etc.	Number Amount Duration Distance Frequency Time	

absent objects or events may increase frequency and variety of questions if paired with games like "Guess What I'm Thinking Of" or "20 Questions." These techniques, of course, are only appropriate for children 3½ years old or older. Diaries of questions asked are recommended for younger children. Usually mothers can generate a fairly complete list in 2 to 3 days of observing and recording.

The general semantic notions requested by Wh-words may be further specified according to the content of the question itself. For example, quality information or descriptions (color, texture, size, shape) may be requested by either *what* questions ("What color is it?") or *how* questions ("How large is it?"). Attitudes, reasons, belief, opinion, and judgment may be requested by *what* or *why* questions, "Why did he lie?", "What do you think will happen next?" Needs and desires may be requested with *what* questions "What do you want?" Many categories can be generated to explore meanings requested. We have found it productive to list the kinds of information requested in the transcript. The relation of these meanings to expectations from the child's cognitive level and structural level of development can then be examined.

There are a variety of intersentence and contextual relations that might be investigated in the speech of clinical populations. These relations could include pronominal reference, deixis, discourse cohesion, and communicative intent to name a few. But since there is very little developmental information in these areas, and because they border so closely on pragmatic questions, we do not attempt to deal with them in this chapter. Some of these issues are discussed in Chapter 4. The others must wait for research that can provide us with data necessary for comparing the performance of clinical populations to that of normal children.

In summary, semantic analyses can include exploration of both referential and relational meanings. Relational meaning can be examined both within and between sentences in conversation. Semantic analyses of speech samples in the clinic are useful for providing information on the diversity and complexity of the concepts and connections children can talk about. They have proved difficult to devise because we lack the data on developmental changes that normally occur in the expression of meaning, and because semantics is so difficult to separate from the cognition on which it is based and the grammatical and pragmatic structures with which it interacts. We have presented a framework for thinking about semantic questions and a few suggestions for devising experimental analysis procedures. The future can only bring improvements in this unfortunate state of affairs.

APPENDIX A
Sample Transcript

Name of child: Mark
Clinic number: ______
Chronological age: 6–8
Date of evaluation: ______
Examiners: ______

Child MLU: 2.50
Number of utterances: 53
Number of intelligible utterances: 52
Sources of transcription: Audiotape

Adult MLU:
1. Mother
2. Clinician
3.

Key:
C = Child
E = Examiner
XXX = unintelligible
. . . = pause

[ ] Gloss or contextual notes
( ) Questionable transcription
/ / Phonetic transcription

Situation variables:
Time of day: 1:30 p.m.
Setting: Waisman Center (Rm. 145)
Materials used: Blocks, puzzle, PAT pictures, DLM pictures, puppet
Length of interaction: 18 minutes
Participants/Type of interactions: 1. Clinician-child
2.
3.
4.

Pragmatics		Speaker	Utterance Number	Dialogue	Morpheme Count		Syntax (see Appendix B)	Semantics (see Table 12)
Child	Adult				Child	Adult		
		C	1.	Hey, that Cookie Monster stands.	5		Regular 3rd person sing. (RTPS)/✓ Stage III, Demon	Demon.Agt.-St.-Expr.
		E		1. That stands? 2. It sure does. 3. Mark, do you know who this is?				
		C	2.	Oscar.	1			Entity (1)
		E		4. Is that Oscar? 5. Or is that the Cookie Monster?				
		C	3.	Oscar.	1			Entity (1)
		E		6. Oscar!				
		C	4.	Cookie Monster in there. [box]	3		in/✓ c. copula/ –	Entity-Locative
		E		7. The Cookie Monster's in there? 8. I thought this was the Cookie Monster?				
		C		(shakes head)				

continued

Pragmatics Child	Pragmatics Adult	Speaker	Utterance Number	Dialogue	Morpheme Count Child	Morpheme Count Adult	Syntax (see Appendix B)	Semantics (see Table 12)
		E		9. This is Oscar?				
				10. Well, thank you for telling me.				
				11. Do you know what Mark?				
				12. This is a special kind of Oscar; he only talks if you ask him questions.				
				13. Do you think you can make Oscar talk?				
				14. Remember, he only talks if you ask him questions.				
				15. You try it, okay?				
				. . .				
				16. I don't hear him talking.				
				17. How about if I try it?				
				. . .				
				18. How are you today Oscar?				
				19. "Just fine thanks, how are you?"				
				20. Fine, I'm pretty good.				
				21. This is my friend Mark over here.				
				. . .				
				22. He's not talking is he?				
				23. We have to ask him a question.				
				24. What could we ask him? [whispering to Mark]				
				25. Mark, you ask him that one.				
				26. Make him talk to you, ask him.				
		C	5. Hi, Oscar.		2			Routine Greeting
		E		27. Good job.				
				28. Now you have to ask him a question.				
				29. What could you ask him?				

		C 6. You like Cookie Monster? E 30. "Oh, I like the Cookie Monster; he's my friend." 31. You made him talk!	3		Stage III, Y/N question	Expr.-St.-Entity
		C 7. Here. [giving Oscar a donut] E 32. He's not going to open his mouth. 33. Maybe we could ask him to open his mouth.	1			Conv. Device: Accompaniment
		C 8. You open your mouth? E 34. There he opened his mouth because you asked him a question. 35. "I don't like green donuts." 36. What do we have to do?	4		Stage III, Y/N question	Agent-Action Possessor-Entity
		C 9. You open your mouth? E 37. "I don't think I like blue donuts." 38. What color is that? 39. Aqua. 40. "I don't like aqua donuts either." 41. What do you want him to do?	4		Stage III, Y/N question	Same as #8
		C 10. Open your mouth. E 42. Did you ask him a question? 43. Ask him again, he didn't hear you.	3			Action-Poss.-Entity
		C 11. Open your mouth. E 44. "Oh, I don't like little blue donuts either." 45. I wonder what else he likes? 46. I wonder what he likes to eat? 47. Why don't you ask him?	3			Same as #10

continued

Pragmatics		Speaker	Utterance Number	Dialogue	Morpheme Count		Syntax (see Appendix B)	Semantics (see Table 12)
Child	Adult				Child	Adult		
		C	12.	You open your mouth.	4			Same as #8
		E	48.	I wonder what he likes to eat?				
		C	13.	Humm, food.	1			Object
		E	49.	I don't know, ask him.				
		C	14.	You like food?	3		Stage III, Y/N question	Exp.-St.-Entity
		E	50.	"I love food."				
			51.	Oscar's not very talk-ative is he?				
			52.	Is there anything else we could ask him?				
			53.	I wonder if he has any friends.				
		C		[sneezes twice]				
		E	54.	Goodness, you have a cold don't you?				
		C	15.	Yeah.	1		Stage III, Y/N question	Con. Device: Affirmation
		E	55.	I wonder if Oscar has any friends.				
		C	16.	You like red?	3			Expr.-St.-Att.
			17.	Open your mouth.	3			Same as #10
		E	56.	"Nope, yuk, I don't like red either."				
		C	18.	We get the Cookie Monster?	4		Stage III, Y/N question *the*/✓	Benef.-Action-Object
		E	57.	Okay, then we can talk to Oscar.				
		C	19.	Where's that? [Cookie Monster]	3		Stage IV, Wh-question c. copula/✓	Location-Entity
		E	58.	Did you see him in there?				
		C	20.	No.	1			Negation (Denial)
		E	59.	You didn't see him in there? . . .				
			60.	Was he here last time you were here?				
		C		Hummmmm.				Conv. Device: Interjection
		E	61.	Oh, that doesn't mean he's still here.				
			62.	I guess we only have Oscar to play with.				
			63.	Do you want to sit down?				
		C	21.	What is that? [cereal]	3		Stage IV, Wh-question c. copula/✓	Entity-Demon.
		E	64.	Yep, let's sit. . .				

		Speaker	Utterance				
		C	22. What is it? [cereal]	3		Stage IV, Wh-question c. copula/✓	Entity-Demon.
		E	65. . . . down at the table, okay?				
		C	23. Hey! Hey!	1			Conv. Device: Interjection
		E	66. Oh, more food for Oscar.				
		C	[Laughs]				
		E	67. [Laughs] Do you have the other food? 68. Mark, sit down. 69. Thank you. 70. Do you think Oscar has any friends?				
		C	24. You like that [cereal], huh? 25. Eat that? [cereal]	4 2		Stage III, Y/N question Stage III, NP Elaboration	Expr.-St.-Demon. Action-Demon.
		E	71. Oh, that was a question! 72. "Yuk, I don't like that either."				
		C	[Laughs]				
		E	73. I wonder what he likes?				
		C	26. Mmmm, you like that? [chips]	3		Stage III, Y/N question	Expr.-St.-Demon.
		E	74. You think he'll like that? [chips] 75. Ask him.				
		C	27. You like that? [chips]	3		Stage III, Y/N question	Same as #26
		E	76. "No, No."				
		C	28. Now my turn.	3		Stage II, NP Elaboration c. copula/ –	Adverbial (A/A) Possessor-Entity
		E	77. Okay, your turn. . . . 78. Now you make him talk if I ask a question. 79. Oscar, do you have any friends?				
		C	29. Yes.	1			Conv. Device: Affirmation
		E	80. Who are your friends? 81. Who are they?				
		C	30. Grover.	1			Entity (1)
		E	82. Grover; who else?				
		C	31. Cookie Monster.	1			Entity (1)
		E	83. Cookie Monster? 84. You like that mean ol' Cookie Monster? 85. Do you like him? 86. Oscar, do you like Cookie Monster?				

continued

Pragmatics		Speaker	Utterance Number	Dialogue	Morpheme Count		Syntax (see Appendix B)	Semantics (see Table 12)
Child	Adult				Child	Adult		
		C	32.	Yes.	1			Conv. Device: Affirmation
		E		87. Doesn't he take all your cookies?				
		C	33.	Yes.	1			Conv. Device: Affirmation
		E		88. Where do you live, Oscar?				
				89. Where do you live?				
		C	34.	Downtown.	1			Locative
		E		90. Downtown on Sesame Street?				
		C	35.	Yes.	1			Conv. Device: Affirmation
		E		91. Let's put Oscar away.				
				92. Can I have him back?				
		C	36.	Hey, what's that? [Points to tape recorder]	4		Stage IV, Wh-question c. copula/✓	Entity-St.-Demon.
				[Activity Change]				
		E		93. What should we make, Mark?				
		C	37.	Hey, neat; look.	3			Conv. Device: Positive Eval. Attention
		E		94. Yeah, see how they [puzzle pieces] fit to-gether?				
		C	38.	Hey, does that bus fit in here? [garage of house]	8		Early IV, Y/N question Stage III, Demon. in/✓ Irregular 3rd person sing./✓	Demon.-Entity-St.-Locative
		E		95. Uh huh.				
		C		Uh huh.				Conv. Device: Affirmation
		E		96. Oh, the bus doesn't fit in.				
		E		97. We can put 'em where?				
		C	39.	Up here.	2			Locative
		E		98. Up there on top of the truck.				
		C	40.	A big cover.	3		Stage III, NP elaboration a/✓	Attribute-Entity
				. . .				
		C	41.	Hey, neat.	2			Conv. Device: Positive Eval.
		E		99. What are you doing?				
				100. What did you make?				
		C	42.	Here.	1			Conv. Device: Accompaniment
		E		101. Okay, I'll carry these. [puzzle pieces]				
				102. Thanks.				

		C	43. Here.	1			Conv. Device: Accompaniment
		E	103. More, all those? [puzzle pieces]				
			104. Okay, got 'em.				
			105. I'll tell you what—				
			106. You carry two, okay?				
		C	44. Two for me . . . go right here. oops!	6		Stage III, NP Elaboration Stage I, VP Elaboration	Quantifier-Recip. Action-Locative
		E	107. Thank you.				
		C	45. Please do that puzzle?	4		Stage III, Demon.	Action-Demon.-(Created) Object
		E	108. You want to do a puzzle?				
		C	46. Yes.	1			Conv. Device: Affirmation
		E	109. Okay; should we sit at the table, Mark?				
		C	47. Yeah.	1			Same as #46
		E	110. It's easier to see.				
		C	48. Yeah.	1			Same as #46
		E	111. What do you call this?				
		C	49. That blocks.	3		plural/✓ c. copula/ – No S-O number Agreem't (Post V)	Demon.-Entity
		E	112. Blocks; boy, did we make a mess.				
		C	50. Hey, what is this?	4		Stage IV, Wh-question c. copula/✓	Entity-St.-Demon.
		C	51. Off?	1		Stage III, Y/N question	
		E	Mmm-mmm				
		C	XXX XXX XXX XXX XXX?	3		Stage I, VP Elaboration Irregular 3rd person sing./✓	Demon.-Action
		E	113. Yep.				
		C	52. That come out.				

APPENDIX B
Criteria for Assigning Structural Stage (ASS): Normal Sequence of Structural Development

Charts (Refer to end of table for definitions of symbols used.)

I. PRODUCTION IN THE SINGLE-WORD UTTERANCE PERIOD

Linguistic Stage	Cognitive Level	Age Range	Development	Example	References
Babbling MLU = 0	Sensorimotor Stage IV	8–12 months	**Precursors** 1. Differentiated cries 2. Syllabic babbling 3. Communication games 4. Attends to objects mom looks at 5. Intentional action 6. Repeats vocalizations upon being imitated	Request, greeting surprise, frustration CVCV *Pat-A-Cake* *Peek-A-Boo* *So-Big*	Ricks, 1975 Menyuk, 1974. Bruner, 1975a + b, 1978 Uzgiris and Hunt, 1975
Early One-Word Pre-Stage I MLU = 0–1.00	Sensorimotor Stage V	10–18 months	**Intentional Communication** *Form:* A. *Performatives* 1. Gesture 2. Gesture + vocalization 3. Gesture + word B. *Single-word utterances* 1. Function words a. few in number b. persist from week to week c. used consistently 2. Names a. few in number b. persist from week to week c. used consistently	Point, show Point + CV or V Point + *mama* *There, no, all gone* *Mama, papa, pet name*	Bates, 1976 Bloom, 1973 Bloom, 1973 *continued*

Linguistic Stage	Cognitive Level	Age Range	Development	Example	References
			3. Substantives: May drop out productively from week to week but comprehension remains (i.e., object labels)	*milk, cup, doggie*	Bloom, 1973
			4. Frequency of communicative attempts: Referential expression infrequent	7 words/hour	Greenfield and Smith, 1976
			Semantic roles encoded		
			1. Announcing	*mama, papa, baby, pet name*	Bloom, 1973
			2. Greeting		
			3. Vocative		
			4. Existence	*there, milk,*	Pea, 1978
			5. Rejection	*no (with force)*	
			Intentions expressed		
			1. Request for object or attention	Child points to object with grasping gestures while vocalizing, *uh, uh*	Bates, 1976
			2. Reject	*Uh* with gesture indicating pushing away or head shake	
			3. Comment	Child points to object vocalizing *uh* or *see*	
			4. Routine	*Hi* and *bye*	Greenfield and Smith, 1976
				Ritualized games, e.g., *Down* as knocks blocks down	Menn and Haselkorn, 1977
			What child encodes with object names		
			1. Object he or she uses or acts on	*milk* (drinks it)	Nelson, 1973
			2. Objects that move and change. (Furniture names not likely; doesn't act on and doesn't move or change)	pet name	
			Productive use of words unlike adult use		
			1. Unsystematic overinclusion: Use of one word for several referents loosely associated	*nenin* for nursing, elbow, food, round, etc.	Clark, 1973

			by the child but unsystematic in adults' eyes. (Beginning of Early Words)		
			2. Under-inclusion: Uses words more narrowly than adults	*fafa* only for flowers in one specific picture	Bloom, 1973
			3. Child only names objects and people that are present unless occurrence is a routine		
Middle One-Word Pre-Stage I MLU = 1.0	Sensorimotor Stage VI	18–20 months	*Form: Single-word utterances*		
			1. Rapid vocabulary increase		
			2. Successive single-word utterances (chained)	*man, coat, hat*	Bloom, 1973 Ingram, 1974 Bloom, 1973
			New semantic roles		
			1. Agent-object relations		
			A. Agent	*mama*	Bloom, 1973 Greenfield and Smith, 1976
			B. Action	*go*	Goldin-Meadow,
			C. Object	*ball, cup*	Seligman and
			D. Recurrence (in requests for actions)	*more, milk*	Gelman, 1976
			E. Cessation	*stop*	Pea, 1978
			F. Disappearance	*all gone*	
			2. Object-object relations (Later)		
			A. Possession	*mine*	Ingram, 1974
			B. Nonexistence	*no, pocket*	Bloom, 1973
			C. Location	*there, ball*	
			New intentions expressed		
			1. Onset of verbal dialogue (Answers some routine questions)	answers speech with speech	Lewis, 1951 Ingram, 1974
			A. Asks a *what's that* question as a routine		
			B. Answers some routine questions	answers *What's that? What does the cow say?*	Ingram, 1974 Dihoff and Chapman, 1977
			C. Increased frequency of talking		Ingram, 1974, 1976
Early Stage I MLU = 1.01–1.49	Sensorimotor Stage VI, Beginning of Preoperations	19–22 months	*Form: A. Onset of two-word utterances*		
			Form: B. Single-word utterances predominate		
			Form: C. Successive single-word utterances	*go. mommy. store.*	Bloom, 1973 Greenfield and Smith, 1976

II. NOUN PHRASE (NP) ELABORATION

Linguistic Stage	Cognitive Level	Age (Predicted)	Development	Example	References
Early & Late Stage I MLU = 1.01–1.99	Late Sensorimotor Stage VI Early Preoperations	19–26 months ± 1 SD = 16–31 months	*Form:* *NP* → *(M)* + N M = class of modifiers *Distribution:* Elaborated NPs only occur alone	a coat my mommy that knee more milk this yours	Brown and Bellugi, 1964 Ingram, 1972
Stage II MLU = 2.00–2.49	Early Preoperations	27–30 months ± 1 SD = 21–35 months	*Form:* *Same as Stage I* *Distribution:* Object position only	*a baby* in *that box* that *a chicken* lookie in *the box*	Chapman, 1978 Brown, 1973 deVilliers and deVilliers, 1973b
Stage III MLU = 2.50–2.99	Early Preoperations	31–34 months ± 1 SD = 24–41 months	*Form:* NP → {(demonstrative) / (article)} + (M) + N 1. Demonstratives include: *this, these, those, that* *2. Articles include: *a* and *the* not used appropriately in all obligatory contexts. 3. Modifiers (M) include: a. Quantifiers: *some, alot, two* b. Possessives: *hers, his, mine* c. Adjectives *Distribution:* Subject NP elaboration appears	That *a blue flower.* Doggie eat *the breakfast.* *A horsie* crying. This *my cup.* That *a dog.* *Horsie* stop.	Brown and Bellugi, 1964

Stage IV MLU = 3.00–3.74	Early Preoperations	35–40 months ± 1 SD = 28–48 months	*Form: NP* → {(demonstrative) / (article) / (M) / (possessive)} + (adjective) + N	I like *these toys.* Put in *the extra* one. I want *some more.* He hit *my truck.*	
			M now includes: *some, something, other, more, two, one, another*		
			Distribution: 1. Subject NP now obligatory, noun or pronoun always appears in subject position	*A horsie* run. *These* my toys.	Ingram, 1972
			2. Elaboration of NP at this stage most frequently realized as one element + N; e.g., article or adjective or demonstrative or possessive.	*A boy* hit *my arm.* *I* want *another piece.*	
Stage V MLU = 3.75–4.50	Late Preoperations	41–46 months ± 1 SD = 35–52	*Form: Same as Stage IV* Number agreement between subject and predicate verb phrase continues to be a problem beyond Stage V	Those *my crayon.*	Cazden, 1968

III. VERB PHRASE (VP) ELABORATION

Linguistic Stage	Cognitive Level	Age (Predicted)	Development	Example	Reference
Stage I MLU = 1.01–1.99	Late Sensorimotor Stage VI Early Preoperations	19–26 months ± 1 SD = 16–31 months	*Main verb:* Unmarked by inflection except occasionally by *-ing.* *Auxiliary:* Doesn't appear *Copula:* No copula present *Verb + Particle:* Occasional use	Mommy go. Baby sleep. That mine. pick up put on	Cazden, 1968 Brown, 1973 De Villiers and de Villiers, 1973b Klima and Bellugi, 1966
Stage II MLU = 2.0–2.49	Early Preoperations	27–30 months ± 1 SD = 21–35 months	*Main verb:* Occasionally marked *Auxiliary:* *1. Present progressive, *-ing,* appears, but *be* is absent. 2. Semi-auxiliary appears, preceding a main verb, but without a noun phrase following it. *Gonna, gotta, wanna, hafta* are analyzed as single morphemes. **Copula:* Appears, may not be marked appropriately for tense and number	He stands. Me playing. Mommy running. I gonna play. Wanna go out. Where's the puppy?	
Stage III MLU = 2.50–2.99	Early Preoperations	31–34 months ± 1 SD = 24–41 months	*Main verb:* 1. Now obligatory *2. Regular past *-ed* overgeneralization begins *Auxiliary:* 1. Present tense auxiliaries appear: *can* *will* **be* (may be incorrectly marked for tense and number. *Am, 'm,* most frequent; *is, 's, are, 're* less frequent.)	Baby eat cookie. Why Paul waked up? I failed that down. He can play. Suzy will come, too. I is going.	Chapman, Paul and Wanska, in preparation
Stage IV MLU = 3.0–3.74	Early Preoperations	35–40 months ± 1 SD = 28–48 months	*Main verb:* *1. Regular past *-ed:* Main verb and auxiliary may be doubly marked for past in negative sentences	I didn't spilled it.	

			Auxiliary: 1. At least one past modal; *could, would, should, must, might;* *2. be + *-ing* appears	I could eat it. We would have two. I should go home. He must sit down. I might like that.	Chapman, Paul, and Wanska, in preparation
			Verb Phrase: Semi-auxiliary complements now take noun phrase	I wanna play ball.	
Stage V MLU = 3.75–4.50	Late Preoperations	41–46 months ± 1 SD = 35–52 months	See "Fourteen Morphemes" (Figure 1)		
Post-Stage V MLU = 4.51 +	Late Preoperations	47 + months ± 1 SD–41 months on	*Main verb/auxiliary:* 1. Past tense *be* appears: *was, were.* 2. *have* + *-en* used infrequently Present tense auxiliary use at Post-Stage V *Distribution:* Percentage of children using each at least once.	He was a silly boy. They were running a race. I have ridden the bus before.	Chapman, Paul, and Wanska, in preparation
			MLU = 4.5–4.99 / MLU = 5.0–5.49 *can* 100% / 100% *will* 71% / 91% *are* 43% / 36% *am* 100% / 91% *is* 71% / 41% N = 7 / N = 11		
			Past modal at Post-Stage V *Distribution:* Percentage of children using each at least once		Chapman, Paul, and Wanska, in preparation
			MLU = 4.5–4.99 / MLU = 5.0–5.49 *would* 14% / 82% *could* 57% / 36% *should* 29% / 45% *must* 43% / 0 *might* 14% / 36% N = 7 / N = 11		

IV. NEGATION

Linguistic Stage	Cognitive Level	Age (Predicted)	Development	Example	References
Stage I through Early Stage II MLU = 1.01–2.24	Late Sensorimotor Stage VI & Early Preoperations	19–28 months ±1 SD = 16–34 months	*Form:* $S \rightarrow \begin{Bmatrix} \text{(no)} \\ \text{(not)} \end{Bmatrix} + \begin{Bmatrix} \text{(NP)} \\ \text{(VP)} \end{Bmatrix}$ or $S \rightarrow (NP + no)$ *No* and *not* are used to negate entire sentence	No night night. No milk. Not go. Daddy no. Ginger no. No hum hum hum (song name) No daddy sit.	Klima and Bellugi, 1966 Chapman, 1978
Late Stage II and Stage III MLU = 2.25–2.99	Early Preoperations	29–34 months ±1 SD = 24–41 months	*Form:* $S \rightarrow NP + (Neg) + VP$ $Neg \rightarrow \begin{Bmatrix} No \\ Not \\ Can't \\ Don't \\ Won't \end{Bmatrix}$ *(Late Stage III* 1. Negative elements now include *no, not, can't,* and *don't* 2. *Can't* and *don't* appear earlier than *can* and *do* and are considered single morphemes, not analyzed as aux. + neg. 3. Negative elements occur after the subject and before the predicate	He no bite you. He can't play. Daddy no bye-bye. Ginger no kiss. Susie don't hit. You can't do that. I won't. It won't move.	Chapman, Paul, and Wanska, in preparation

Early Stage IV MLU = 3.0–3.49	Early Preoperations	35–38 months ± 1 SD = 28–45 months	*Form:* *Aux* → *C* + V^{aux} + *(Neg)* *C* → *Tense & number marker* V^{aux} {*can*, *will*, *do*, *be*}	I'm not going. He can't play. He is not. He can not play. I will not play.	Chapman, Paul, and Wanska, in preparation
			1. *Can't* and *don't* now analyzed as *aux* + *(neg)*, two morphemes, e.g., *can not, do not*	He doesn't have it. He does not play ball. Susie won't kiss him. I don't want it. That isn't going fast.	
			2. Auxiliary elements, contracted or uncontracted, can include: present tense *be, can, do, did, does,* and *will.*	This isn't mine. There aren't any more. He doesn't sit down. They won't play. We didn't go outside.	
Late Stage V MLU = 4.0–4.49	Late Preoperations	43–46 months ± 1 SD = 37–52 months	1. Auxiliary elements contracted or uncontracted now include: past tense *be* and past tense modals	He shouldn't be eating. George wasn't home. They weren't in school.	Chapman, Paul, and Wanska, in preparation
			2. Past tense contracted *be* and past tense modals appear infrequently, e.g., *wasn't, wouldn't, couldn't, shouldn't.*	I couldn't fix that toy. He wouldn't help me.	

V. YES/NO QUESTIONS

Linguistic Stage	Cognitive Level	Age (Predicted)	Development	Example	References
Stages I, II, and III MLU = 1.01–2.99	Late Sensorimotor Stage IV and Early Preoperations	19–34 months ± 1 SD = 16–41 months	Marked only by rising intonation	Mommy see? See hole? No ear? See my doggie? You can't fix it? That block too?	Klima and Bellugi, 1966 Chapman, Paul, and Wanska, in preparation
Early Stage IV MLU = 3.0–3.49	Early Preoperations	35–38 months ± 1 SD = 28–45 months	1. Auxiliary begins to be used and is appropriately inverted	Am I silly? It can't be a bigger truck? Can't it be a bigger truck? Do I look like a baby?	
			2. Auxiliary elements include present tense *be, can, will,* and *do*	Is he going too? Will he bring it home?	
			3. Rising intonation continues to be an alternative form for asking yes/no questions	Can I go in the playpen? Can I talk to grandma again? You want to go out? Wanna talk to mama? Want some birthday cake? Wanna see it? Wanna go out?	

VI. Wh-QUESTIONS

Linguistic Stage	Cognitive Level	Age (Predicted)	Development	Example	References
Stage I and Early Stage II MLU = 1.01–2.24	Late Sensorimotor Stage VI and Early Preoperations	19–28 months ± 1 SD = 16–34 months	*Routine forms of Wh-questions:*		
			1. *What* {(this) / (that)} ?	What this? What that?	Klima and Bellugi, 1966
			2. *What* (NP) *do(ing)*?	What you do? What he doing?	Ervin-Tripp, 1970 Chapman, Paul, and Wanska, in preparation
			3. *Where* (NP) *go(ing)*?	Where the ball go? Where daddy going?	
Late Stage II MLU = 2.25–2.49	Early Preoperations	29–30 months ± 1 SD = 24–35 months	*Novel Wh-questions appear:*		
			1. *What* + (N) + V	What getting? What you eat?	
			2. *Where* + (N) + V	Where he going? What he do there?	
Stage III MLU = 2.50–2.99	Early Preoperations	31–34 months ± 1 SD = 24–41 months	*Auxiliary:* Begins to appear but is *not inverted.*	Why I can't go?	Tyack and Ingram, 1977
			Frequent Wh-words include: *what, what doing, where*	Where the glass of milk is?	
			Infrequent Wh-words include: *why, who,* and *how*	Who it is? Why you hit me?	
Early Stage IV MLU = 3.0–3.49	Early Preoperations	35–42 months ± 1 SD = 28–45 months	*Auxiliary:*		
			1. Appropriately inverted at least once	Where is the glass of milk? Who is that? Why is he running?	Chapman, Paul, and Wanska, in preparation
			2. Auxiliary elements include: Present tense *be, can, will,* and *do.*	Why don't you like stamps on it?	
			Wh-words: *When* questions appear	When is he going?	

Developed by Jon F. Miller and Robin S. Chapman

*Structures at the emergence level in this chart appear at the mastery level in the 14 morpheme analysis.

→ is expanded, or elaborated, as

{x / y / z} only one item within the brackets can occur

{(x) / (y) / (z)} either one of the items, or none, can occur

(x) the item within the braces is optional. It may or may not occur.

APPENDIX C
Complex Sentence Development

STAGE: Early IV **MLU: 3.00–3.50** **PREDICTED AGE: 34–37 MONTHS** **NUMBER OF CHILDREN IN GROUP (N) = 16**

	Development		
Section	**Reached by 50%–90% of children**	**Reached by over 90% of children**	**Example**
1		Percent of TRUE complex sentences (excluding those containing catenatives: *gonna, wanna, gotta, hafta, s'posedta, let's,* and *let me*) in a 15-minute speech sample is between 1% and 10%. Both conjoined and embedded sentences are included.	When calculating percentage of complex sentences: *EXCLUDE* sentences like: The car's *gonna* crash. I *wanna* go home. We *gotta* work fast. I don't *hafta* play. *Let's* play fish.
2	*Simple infinitive clauses (not unanalyzed catenatives listed in #1) with subjects that are the same as that of the main sentence. The subject of the clause is usually deleted.		He *has to move.* She *wants to get out.* *Try to brush* her hair. Daddy *wanted to wear* shorts. He *likes to bite.* I *need to go.*
	Sentences containing *let's* or *let me*		*Let's* get in. *Let me* see.
	*Sentences containing full propositional complements, headed by verbs like *think, guess, wish, wonder, know, hope, show, remember, pretend, forget.* The clause may or may not be marked by *that.*		The doctor says *that baby's crying.* I think *we have some here.* Pretend *you said it.* You mean *the scooper goes* back of the bulldozer?
	*Sentences containing simple non-infinitive Wh-clause marked by *what, where, why, how, if,* etc.		I know *what we could play.* Look *how big I am.* Remember *where it is?*
3	*Sentences with two clauses conjoined		*Then it broke* and *we didn't have it anymore.*
4	*Conjunction *and*		Then it broke *and* we didn't have it anymore.
5	Number of different conjunctions $\overline{X} = 2$, ± 1 SD $= 0–4$		

STAGE: Late IV–Early V **MLU: 3.51–4.00** **PREDICTED AGE: 38–42 MONTHS** **(N) = 15**

	Development		
Section	**Reached by 50%–90% of children**	**Reached by over 90% of children**	**Example**
1		Percent of TRUE complex sentences: 1%–10%.	
2	*Sentences containing more than one embedding (One of the clauses may include a catenative)		The tea is *gonna start to fall.* I *think* we *gotta pour* some lemon in it.
3	*Sentences containing both a conjoined and embedded clause (One may be a catenative)		It's *not a bulldozer,* ***'cause*** *it don't have something* ***to scoop.*** *He wants* ***to stay at his home today,*** and *I don't know why.*
4	No new conjunctions		
5	$\underline{N}$umber of different conjunctions $\bar{X} = 3$, ± 1 SD $= 1$–5		

STAGE: Late V **MLU: 4.01–4.50** **PREDICTED AGE: 43–46 MONTHS** **(N) = 13**

Section	Development: Reached by 50%–90% of children	Development: Reached by over 90% of children	Example
1	Percent of TRUE complex sentences: 10%–20%.		
2	†Sentences containing infinitive clauses with subjects different from that of main sentence		This is the way *to do it.* I want *it to go* chug-chug. Daddy made this *for me to sit on.* I can't get *this thing to move.*
	Sentences containing relative clauses (They may or may not contain *that* or *which*)		This kind is not the kind *that I like.* They're boys *what you know.* Where are the tracks *that belong to this?*
		Sentences containing full propositional clauses	I know *that we have some.* I think *we should go home.* Pretend *you said it.*
		Sentences containing simple non-infinitive Wh-clauses	I know *what we could play.* Remember *where it is?*
		Sentences containing more than one embedding. (One may be a catenative)	I *think we gotta* **pour some lemon in it.**
3		Sentences with two clauses conjoined.	*Then it broke,* and *we didn't have it anymore.*
4	*Conjunction *if*		We always go outside, *if* it's not raining.
5	Number of different conjunctions, $\overline{X} = 4$, ±1 SD = 2–6		

STAGE: V + **MLU: 4.51-5.00** **PREDICTED AGE: 47 + MONTHS** **(N) = 8**

Section	Development: Reached by 50%-90% of children	Development: Reached by over 90% of children	Example
1	Percent of TRUE complex sentences: 10%-20%		
2	†Sentences containing gerund (-ing) clauses [Note: gerunds used as adjectives are not counted. The following sentences are *not* complex: These are *running* shoes. I have a *fishing* rod. The *stacking* cups are red.]		I felt like *turning it.* We could make it start *working* with this. Go *fishing.* They'll hear us *talking on the recorder.*
	†Sentences containing Wh-infinitive clauses		You know *how to make one.* I don't know *where to put the neck.* Show me *what to do.*
	Sentences containing unmarked infinitive clauses headed by *help, make, watch, let*		She made *him talk today.* Help *me pick these up.* I'll let *it go now.* Watch *me jump.*
		Sentences containing simple infinitive clauses with subjects the same as that of the main sentence	She wants *to get out.* Daddy likes *to wear shorts.*
3	No new forms of conjoining		
4	Conjunction *because*		This car is winning, *'cause* he's got the faster horn.
		Conjunction *and*	Then it broke, *and* we didn't have it anymore.
5	Number of different conjunctions, $\overline{X} = 4$, ± 1 SD = 2–6		

STAGE: V + + **MLU: 5.01-up** **PREDICTED AGE: 47 + MONTHS** **(N) = 7**

Section	Development: Reached by 50%-90% of children	Development: Reached by over 90% of children	Example
1	Percent of TRUE complex sentences: over 20%		
2	No new forms of embedding		
3		Sentences containing both a conjoined and an embedded clause	*He wants* ***to stay at his home today*** and *I don't know why.*
4	Conjunctions *when* and *so*		I can get the train out *when* it's like this. Let me close the gate *so* it won't come out.
		Conjunction *if*	We always go outside, *if* it's not raining.
5	Number of different conjunctions $\overline{X} = 7$, ±1 SD = 6–8		

Developed by Rhea Paul.
*These forms appear at a later stage, indicating use by 90% of subjects in a higher MLU group.
†Although the use of the clause increased with MLU, the increase was not statistically significant.

CHAPTER 3

A Comparison of Six Structural Analysis Procedures: *A Case Study*

Thomas M. Klee and Rhea Paul

Contents

The speech-language clinician has a number of formal procedures available for analyzing a sample of spontaneous language. These procedures are generally used to determine the nature and extent of any delay present in the child's productive language system. Such a determination is usually made by describing the child's linguistic system and assessing its status relative to that of other children of similar chronological or mental age. Depending, of course, on the child's particular problems, such a description may involve evaluating one or more aspects of production: phonological, semantic, syntactic, or pragmatic. But the majority of formal analysis procedures have only concerned themselves with syntax, and it is to syntax alone that we, too, address ourselves. Syntactic analysis procedures involve parsing each utterance into its constituents and analyzing the grammatical forms and constructions present in it. Each construction is then assigned to a developmental stage, which is derived from research on normal children. By examining the range of stages present in a transcript, a concomitant language-age level is usually assigned. This information is then used to characterize the general nature of the child's linguistic system (i.e., is the child using various forms of language characteristic of younger normal children, or is he or she using idiosyncratic forms?) and to determine the existence and degree of language delay.

A second purpose of language analysis is to develop appropriate goals for intervention, should the diagnosis indicate that remediation is warranted. These goals are usually established by comparing the child's present level of functioning with that of normally developing children of similar chronological or mental age and identifying areas of grammatical discrepancy. These areas are targeted for remediation. The precision of the analytic tool is important, since it is not only used for description and diagnosis but also as a basis for educational planning.

The choice of procedure for grammatical analysis has not ordinarily been thought to be of great importance. Clinicians often simply choose one of the standard tools, develop a familiarity with it, and use it consistently. The assumption underlying this practice has been that the various systems of analysis really yield the same information, and the choice of one over another is merely a matter of personal preference.

The aim of this case study is to put that assumption to the test. By applying six of the most widely used analysis procedures to the grammar of one speech sample, it is possible to determine whether, in fact, all procedures yield the same general stage assignment and provide descriptive detail comparable in amount, quality, and focus. It is also possible to compare the analyses in terms of clinical efficiency. In addition to the comparison of the results of the analyses, we have also established a set of desirable features by which each of the procedures was rated. The goal has not been to choose the one "best" method but to identify the differences among them.

In addition to the six standard analyses, a grammar based on a transformational model was also written for the speech sample. We believed the grammar would provide the greatest amount of detail against which we could compare results of the other procedures. The intent here is not to suggest grammar writing as an alternative form of speech sample analysis in the clinic. In fact, this analysis is rather poorly suited to clinical purposes because it yields no age equivalent and because few normative data exist for comparative purposes. The detailed grammar will be used instead to illuminate the strengths and weaknesses of the other tools. The purpose of this grammar is to *describe* the child's language production; no attempt has been made to ensure that the proposed grammar is in any way "psychologically real."

CASE DESCRIPTION

Jay is a 3-year, 5-month-old boy who had attended a preschool educational program for 7 months at the time of his evaluation. His teacher referred him for an assessment primarily because of her difficulties in understanding his speech. The teacher reported, however, that Jay was "cognitively more advanced" than most of his classroom peers and that he adjusted quickly and easily to the social/academic environment of the classroom.

As part of a comprehensive communication evaluation, four measures of language comprehension were used. The Miller-Yoder Test of Grammatical Comprehension (Miller and Yoder, 1972), which requires a discriminative pointing response to a set of four pictures, showed Jay to be functioning at a 4-year-old level on all items, with the exception of pronoun comprehension. On a test of single-word receptive vocabulary, the Peabody Picture Vocabulary Test (Dunn, 1965), Jay's score fell at the 64th percentile, which is equivalent to a "vocabulary age" of 3;10. On two informal comprehension tests, the Bellugi-Klima object manipulation task (Bellugi-Klima, 1968) and a Wh-question task (Chapman, in preparation), Jay's performance was at age level.

Jay performed above age level by approximately 8-12 months on two measures of cognitive development. On the Slosson Intelligence Test for Children (Slosson, 1974) Jay's mental age (MA) was 4;5. On the McCarthy Scales of Children's Abilities (McCarthy, 1972) Jay's MA was 4;3. (This later test was given when Jay was 3;7).

Because Jay's mental age was not depressed relative to his chronological age, we can expect Jay's linguistic development to be synchronous with chronological age. Had his CA exceeded his MA, indicating a cognitive delay, our criterion would have shifted to judging linguistic development relative to cognitive status.

In summary, both Jay's cognitive level and his level of linguistic comprehension appear at or above expectations for his chronological age.

THE ANALYSIS PROCEDURES

Six standard structural analysis procedures were applied to a 30-minute free-speech sample recorded on audiotape while Jay played with toys and talked with a clinician. Five of the procedures are "structural" in the sense that they analyze utterances into constituents that are then classified according to their order of emergence in normal acquisition.

These analyses do not, however, specify the hierarchical relations among constituents. For example, a noun phrase (NP) might consist of an adjective, a noun, or a prepositional phrase. That prepositional phrase might, itself, be broken down into a preposition and another NP. The procedures do not incorporate these relationships. Nor do they demonstrate the child's capacity to form stylistic variants (transformations) of base sentences. The grammar written for comparison with the standard procedures provides a finely detailed description of the language sample. It also points out hierarchical relations and stylistic flexibility within the system. However, it has the rather colossal disadvantage of offering no means for comparing the sample with developmental norms.

A brief description of each of the analyses performed on Jay's sample of spontaneous language follows. Procedural aspects of each of the systems is kept to a minimum, since it is assumed the reader has some familiarity with the specifics of sampling, analyzing, and scoring required by each. The discussion focuses instead on the diagnosis of Jay's productive language that each analysis provides.

The transcript on which the analyses are based is found in the chapter appendix, pages 99-110.

Mean Length of Utterance

Mean length of utterance (MLU) in morphemes (Brown, 1973) is a general index of grammatical development and has been shown to increase with age up to MLUs of 4.00-4.50. De Villiers and de Villiers' (1973a) modification of Brown's five original stages resulted in equal stage intervals of 0.50 morphemes for each of five stages, ranging from 1.00-3.49 morphemes and a sixth stage ranging from 3.50-4.25. Miller and Chapman (pages 25-27) modified this further and established age ranges for each of eight stages (0.50 morphemes per stage) based on 123 normally developing children ranging in age from 17 months to 59 months. From this, two linear regression equations were derived. One predicts MLU given age; the other, age given MLU.

Based on the 167 utterances in Jay's language sample, an MLU of 3.08 was calculated using the rules specified by Brown (1973). This is characteristic of Miller and Chapman's Early Stage IV (35-38 months). Using the Miller and Chapman data, an MLU of 3.08 would predict an age equivalent of 35.0 months, approximately 6 months below Jay's actual age. Given that Jay is 41 months of age, his predicted MLU would be 3.67, or 0.61 morphemes higher than that found in the sample.

When attempting to determine if a particular MLU is within normal limits of development for a given age, a measure of variability is necessary. Miller and Chapman have calculated standard deviations from both predicted age and predicted MLU. Jay's MLU of 3.08 falls within one standard deviation from the mean value predicted for his chronological age. At 41 months of age the predicted MLU range at ± 1 SD is 2.87-4.47. Based on MLU alone Jay appears within normal limits with regard to general syntactic development (see Figure 3).

The computation of Jay's MLU was derived by a close adherence to Brown's rules (1973, p. 54). However, when attempting to analyze the grammatical system of a child whose language has advanced past the early stages of development, as has Jay's, it becomes obvious that Brown's counting rules are neither comprehensive nor reflective of the child's advancing syntactic system. That is, the clinician is left with the dilemma of making rather arbitrary morpheme assignments to a number of ambiguous grammatical items. It becomes apparent that one's decision as to what morpheme value to ascribe to a given construction should be based not only on grammatical constituents (i.e., the number of free and bound morphemes), but must be based in part on semantic and phonological considerations.

The use to which an MLU count is to be put determines which method of computation should be used. If one's intention is to use MLU to make a structural stage assignment using Brown's (1973) stages, one is restricted to using Brown's counting rules (1973, p. 54). Alteration or modification of those counting rules would invalidate assigning a structural stage of development to the child's language. However, if one's intention is to attempt to account for the child's morpho-syntactic system in terms of which morphemes are "psychologically real" for the child, the following addenda to Brown's original rules may be considered. Again, use of these modified counting rules necessarily precludes assignment to Brown's stages (1973, p. 56). Because we wished to assign Jay's language sample to a specific developmental stage, we adhered to the original rules.

Compound words present an interesting example of the inadequacies of Brown's counting rule #5:

> All compound words (two or more free morphemes), proper names, and ritualized reduplications count as single words. Examples: *birthday, rackety-boom, choo-choo, quack-quack, night-night, pocketbook, seesaw.* Justification is that no evidence that the constituent morphemes function as such for these children (1973, p. 54).

Essentially, Brown is arguing that multi-morpheme credit should be withheld since there is no a priori evidence that the child is capable of producing the constituent free morphemes that make up a compound word. However, at some point in the child's development, the child's construction and interpretation of his lexicon becomes "adult-like." That is, the systems of children and adults approach parity.

To illustrate this point, Jay's language sample contains instances of the compound word *fireman,* as well as the constituent free morphemes *fire* and *man.* If Jay had provided no productive exemplars in his discourse of either constituent morpheme, we should feel safe, if not conservative, in classifying *fireman* as one morpheme, assuming like Brown, that this compound word served a labeling function only.

Further evidence for double-morpheme credit may be found in the phonological realizations of the word. Jay's production of this word is [fa͜ɪrmæn], unlike the standard adult form [fa͜ɪrmən], indicating he is conjoining two separate morphemes.[1]

Similar rationale may be invoked for other words comprised of two conjoined morphemes. For example, in order to credit a word with two-morpheme status, there must be evidence in the child's language sample (or collateral productive data, if available) that each constituent has been used independently. Otherwise, credit of one-morpheme is justified. This counting rule obtains for negated verbs, reflexive pronouns, and certain phonological alterations such as catenative+infinitive (e.g., *wanna go*).

Let us take the case of judging morpheme (constituent) status for the catenative verbs. Brown's counting rule #8 states:

> Count as separate morphemes. . .all catenatives. These. . .count as single morphemes rather than as *going to* or *want to* because evidence is that they function so for the children (1973, p. 54).

Again, the question must be asked, at what point in development does the child's use of a syntactic construction function as the adult's? From a structural point of view, the answer is at the time the child demonstrates production capacity to generate the constituent morphemes independently. For example, in the adult's lexicon, we evaluate the construction *gonna go* as being composed of four morphemes (cf, *go+ing+to+go*). Yet the older child is given credit for only two morphemes, according to Brown's rule #8. We feel the conservative estimate is justified only in the case of the child at an earlier stage of development, one not evidencing any of the constituent morphemes in production.

The case of diminutives in the older child deserves comment. Brown states in counting rule #7:

> Count as one morpheme all diminutives *(doggie, mommie)* because these children at least do not seem to use the suffix productively. . . (1973, p. 54).

However, it must be recognized that some children (at least) *do* use the suffix productively. For example, if a child produces both *dog* and *doggie,* the suffix results in a distinct phonological form, although this does not alter the semantic representation of the item. Furthermore, because diminutive forms are often among the earliest words to emerge in the child's lexicon (e.g., *mommy, daddy, doggie,* etc.), and because the bound morpheme /i/ does not alter the morphological structure of the word (only the phonological) in the direction of greater complexity, we take the tack that this phonological epenthesis is undeserving of separate morpheme credit. In sum, we agree with Brown's original decision, albeit with a different rationale.

In conclusion, one's decision rules for assigning values of morpho-syntactic complexity to a child's utterances must change as the child changes. This continual adjustment of the assessment procedure

---

[1]It is interesting to note, however, that [fa͜ɪrman] might be the later ontogenetic phonological form, being closer to the adult form.

should better reflect the child's gradual progression from a child-to-adult linguistic system, viewing development as a continual rather than a discrete process. The caveat that must be kept in mind at the outset of choosing between MLU computations is that the method of computation should be dependent on the use to which the data will be put.

Assigning Structural Stage

The Assigning Structural Stage (ASS) procedure is described in detail in Chapter 2. A worksheet that can be used to record data for ASS is shown in Table 1. Each grammatical form from the developmental charts is listed by stage. The language sample is then scanned utterance by utterance, and the constituents within an utterance are noted. Correct usage of a particular constituent is logged in the appropriate column on the worksheet. Examples of attempts that result in incorrect form are logged in the adjacent column.

As Table 1 reveals, Jay's use of syntactic structures ranges from Stage I to Stage V with the greatest portion of structures representing Stages II, III, and IV. Two different stage assignments can be calculated in this analysis. The first is based on frequency of structures produced at each stage and provides an index of mastery for those structures occurring in the transcript. The second method provides an index of acquisition by identifying the most complex utterances of each structural type regardless of frequency. We expect the distribution of structural types across stages to range at least one stage above and below the most frequent stage. Using MLU as the overall indicator, we would expect most of the structural types in Jay's speech to center in Early Stage IV. Miller suggests using this relation between MLU and structural analysis to decide whether a child is delayed or deviant.

Using the first method of stage determination, the mastery criterion, Jay's level of development would be between Stage III and Early Stage IV. The age equivalent for this level of development is estimated to be 35 months of age (Miller, Chapter 2, this volume), and in this case is similar to the MLU assignment. Jay produces few structures above this level, so no stage of emergence can be assigned.

14 Grammatical Morphemes

The 14 grammatical morphemes studied by Brown (1973) and by de Villiers and de Villiers (1973b) are scored in Jay's transcript. The number of obligatory contexts and number of realizations for each of the following morphemes were counted:

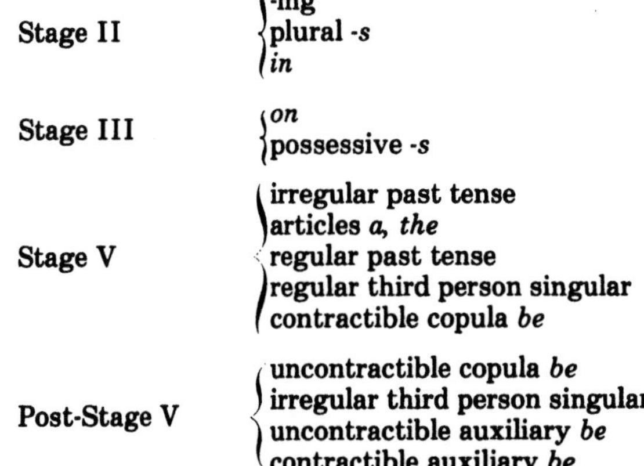

Stage II	-ing plural *-s* *in*
Stage III	*on* possessive *-s*
Stage V	irregular past tense articles *a, the* regular past tense regular third person singular contractible copula *be*
Post-Stage V	uncontractible copula *be* irregular third person singular uncontractible auxiliary *be* contractible auxiliary *be*

The percentage of realizations in obligatory contexts was then computed for each form. The criterion for rule acquisition was 90% correct usage in obligatory contexts. The worksheet for this analysis is shown in Figure 1.

Jay's sample reveals 100% correct usage of all Stage II items. One Stage III item does not appear, the other is 50% correct. Stage V items show variability; some reach 90%, others do not. All Post-Stage V forms except one instance of uncontractible copula are correct less than 90% of the time. Jay's performance falls between Stages III and V by this analysis. This finding corroborates the general stage placement found using both MLU and ASS.

Developmental Sentence Analysis

The Developmental Sentence Score (DSS) (Lee, 1974) is another procedure often used in evaluating a language sample. In deriving a DSS, 50 utterances from the sample are scored. Usually the last 50 consecutive utterances are analyzed to allow for a "warming-up period." Only utterances that contain both a subject and verb are included in the DSS analysis, although less complete utterances can be analyzed using a related procedure, Developmental Sentence Types (DST). Only intelligible, nonimitative and different utterances are included in the analysis.

The DSS divides utterances and their constituents into eight grammatical categories: indefinite and personal pronouns, primary and secondary verbs, negation, conjunctions, interrogative reversals, and Wh-questions. Each of these categories is broken down into eight developmental levels, and a developmental score is assigned to each construction. Those lexical items and grammatical structures that emerge early in the development of the child's language production earn fewer points; those developed later earn a greater number of points. An additional category awards a "sentence point" for each utterance that meets all *adult* standard grammatical

Table 1. Assigning Structural Stage: Summary Worksheet

	Syntactic structure	Structural stage	Utterance number	Examples of attempts,[a] or omission in obligatory context
II.	Noun Phrase Elaboration			
	Plural /s/	II	77	84
	Demonstratives: *this, that, these, those*	III	1, 4, 6, 7, 15, 24, 25, 26, 34, 37, 43, 45B, 47, 48, 53, 54, 55, 56, 57, 58, 60, 61, 64, 75, 80, 83, 84, 92, 97, 99, 113, 116	26
	Quantifiers: *some, alot, two*	III	43	
	one, more, other, another	IV	27, 96, 98	
	Possessives: /s/, *her*(s), *his, mine, my*	III	67, 103, 107	11, 69
	their(s), *our*(s)	IV		
	Adjectives	III	85, 99	
	S-V agreement (number)	Post-V		
	Mod + Adj + N	IV	100	
III.	Verb Phrase Elaboration			
	Main V unmarked	I		4, 6, 7, 11, 24, 34, 35, 74, 95, 99, 107, 111
	V + particle	I	101	
	Semi-aux + V	II	101, 108, 117, 118	
	Copula appears	II	14, 25, 61, 79, 81, 84, 85, 89, 92	
	Aux appears	III	76, 90, 113	75
	Can, will, be (present)	III	39, 86, 105	
	Regular past *-ed* overgeneralization	III		33
	Semi-aux + V + NP	EIV	19, 48, 62, 72, 110, 115	
	Past modals: *could, would, should, must, might*	IV	104	
IV.	Negation			
	No, not used to negate	I, EII		
	NP + (Neg) + VP (Neg ⟶ *no, not, can't, don't, won't*)	LII, III	10, 22, 31, 49, 50, 51, 71, 88, 94, 112	
	isn't, aren't, doesn't	EIV	15, 97	
	wasn't, weren't, wouldn't, couldn't, shouldn't	V		
V.	Yes/No Questions			
	Rising intonation only	I-III	12, 20, 55, 57, 64, 80, 81a	
	Aux inverted	EIV	41a	
VI.	Wh-Questions			
	What {this / that} ?	I, EII	56	
	What (NP) do(ing)?	I, EII		
	Where (NP) go(ing)?	I, EII		
	{What / Where} + Nucleus?	LII	33, 47, 53, 116	
	Wh + Aux (Aux not inverted)	III	58	
	Aux inverted at least once	EIV	1, 3,	60, 78
	When appears	EIV	1,	
VII.	Complex Sentence Development			
	Let me	EIV	65	
	Simple infinitival clause	EIV	90, 106	
	Simple Wh-clause	EIV		
	Double-embedding	LIV-EV		
	Conjoin + embed	LIV-EV		
	Infinitive clause with different subject	LV		
	Relative clause	LV		
	Gerund	V+		
	Wh-infinitive	V+		
	Unmarked infinitive	V+		

[a]"Attempt" signifies syntactic structure is marked, but incorrect by adult standards.

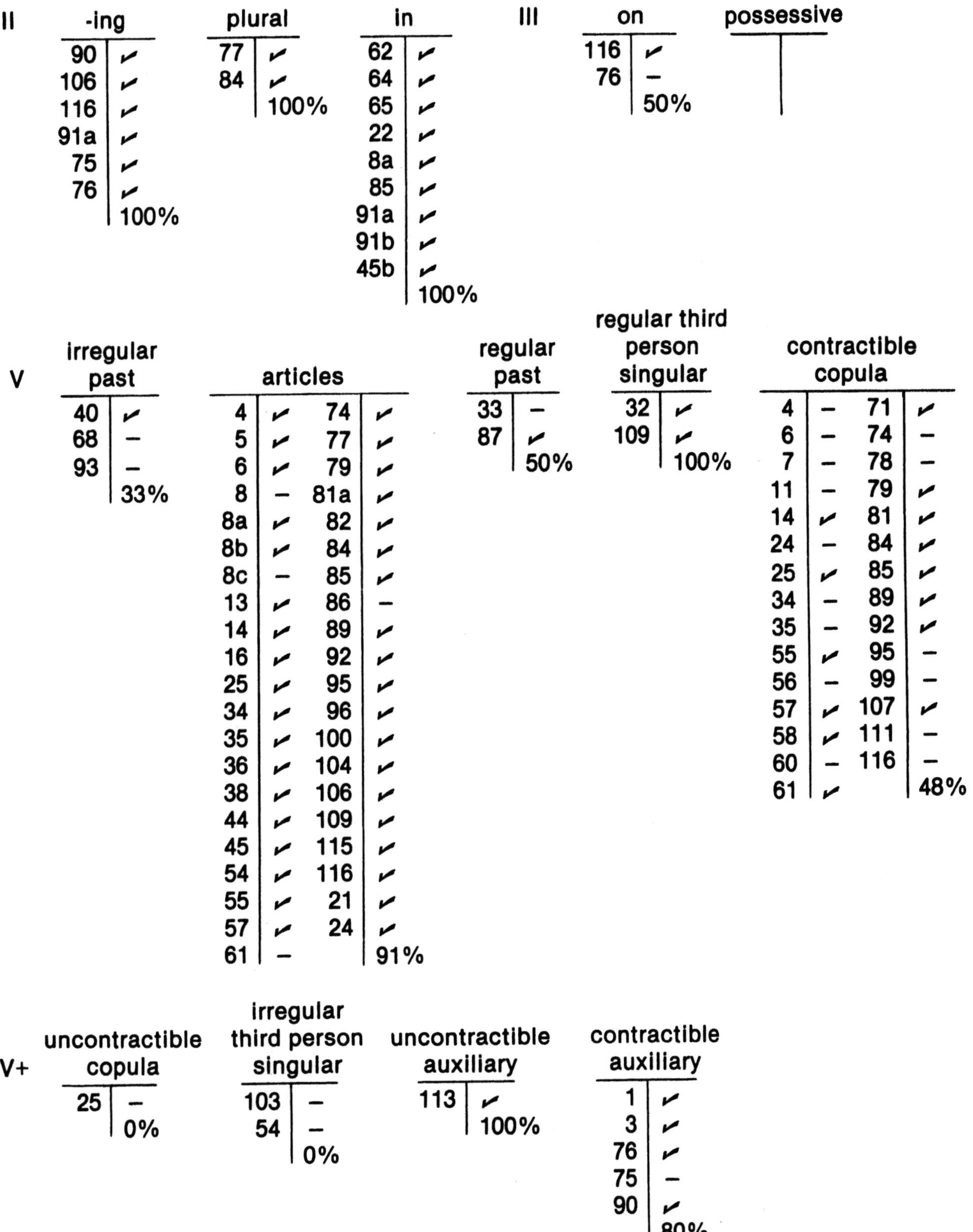

Figure 1. 14 grammatical morpheme analysis. (Morpheme correctly appearing is indicated by (✓); morpheme absent in obligatory context is indicated by (–). Numbers refer to utterance identification from transcript.)

rules. Lee (1974, p. 137) states that this sentence point "is at least a gesture toward acknowledging that there are many more grammatical forms to be considered than the eight categories on the DSS."

A DSS of 4.20 was computed for Jay's sample. This score falls below the 10th percentile for children 41 months of age, indicating that Jay may be a candidate for language intervention. (Of course, collateral assessment data must also be considered in making this decision.) Jay demonstrates a range of developmental levels in all eight DSS categories, but most scores fall in the first and second DSS levels, indicating somewhat limited and immature forms, relative to his age. This is especially characteristic of his use of indefinite and personal pronouns. Jay gets many "attempt" marks in the primary verb category, indicating copula and auxiliary verb omissions as well as inappropriate verb tense and number agreement. Only seven instances of secondary verbs are noted. Finally, Wh-questions are limited to *what* and *where,* with 3 out of 6 instances of failure to invert subject and verb in question forms. Jay earned 26 out of a possible 50 sentence points, indicating he is using sentences that meet adult grammatical standards about half the time. The DSS analysis of Jay's transcript is shown in Table 2.

Language Assessment, Remediation, and Screening Procedure

The Language Assessment, Remediation, and Screening Procedure (LARSP), developed by Crystal, Fletcher, and Garman (1976), describes the child's productive language from a structuralist orientation. But as the authors point out, this "does not preclude using certain transformational notions; indeed, the grammatical framework on which (this) approach is based frequently incorporates them" (p. 35). The child's language system is segmented for analysis into four levels of structural organization: sentence, clause, phrase, and word types.

Use of the LARSP requires eight scans of the transcript to complete the analysis of the four grammatical levels. The first scan determines the range of sentences that can be analyzed. The second scan establishes the proportion of spontaneous sentences to response sentences. Scan 3 analyzes the level of sentence connectivity. Scan 4 surveys utterances for coordination, subordination, etc. Scan 5 analyzes clause structure (e.g., subject, verb, complement, etc.) and the range of constructional types established (SV, SVA, etc.). Scan 6 analyzes phrase structure (e.g., NP, VP, etc.). Scan 7 analyzes word-structure patterns (e.g., bound morphemes). And finally, Scan 8 attempts to clarify "problem" utterances identified in Scan 1 (Crystal et al., 1973, pp. 94–98). Information form these scans is then summarized by frequency counts on the Profile Chart in the LARSP handbook (see Figure 2).

Analysis of Jay's production shows the majority of his clause level types to be within LARSP's Stage III (2;0–2;6 years), with some evidence of emerging clausal constructions in Stage IV (2;6–3;0 years). However, developmentally immature clause types characterizing Stage II development continue to occur, as expected, indicating Jay shows a range of constructions across at least three stages of development. Similar conclusions can be drawn about the phrase level of construction.

Elaboration of the noun phrase, verb phrase, and adverbial phrase at least through Stage IV is evident, indicating growing complexity in expansion at this level of sentence structure. For example, Jay uses 14 utterances classified as XY+C/O: NP (Stage IV). This indicates utterances that have either a complement or object which expands as a noun phrase, along with two other elements of clause structure (e.g., a subject and verb).

Data for some phrase and word level constructions are summarized on the LARSP worksheet, using frequency-of-occurrence information for each structure. This gives the clinician no impression of the proportion of correct realization of forms in obligatory context. For example, Jay's profile chart notes five occurrences of the copula (Stage III), but neglects to inform how many instances of obligatory contexts for this structure exist.

LARSP handles this "problem" by use of an "error box" at Stage VI. At this point in the profile chart, the developmental summary is directed to an analysis of the child's "errors" (which, as Crystal (1979, p. 97) points out, indicate "sign(s) of development, not of failure"). The apparent problem is resolved then, by counting the number of copulas omitted from obligatory contexts, for example, and noting them in the Stage VI error box under *Other.* Crystal (1979, 96ff) cautions that the "negative features" listed at Stage VI are invoked only when there is independent evidence in the language sample that the particular grammatical feature has begun to be acquired. In Jay's case, the copula form has begun to emerge (Stage III: Cop 5) but has not developed into consistent adult-like usage (Stage VI: –Cop 13), and this aspect of his development is reflected in the LARSP profile (Crystal, personal communication, 1980).

Language Sampling, Analysis, and Training

The Language Sampling, Analysis, and Training (LSAT) procedure (Tyack and Gottsleben, 1974), unlike the tools used so far, does not yield an age-equivalent score. Instead, it provides the clinician with a set of baseline data and a group of constructions to be used in establishing therapy goals. A sample size of 100 utterances is suggested for analysis. After scoring each sentence for number of words and morphemes, a word-morpheme index is computed, which is an average of words/sentence and morphemes/sentence measures. One-word/one-morpheme utterances are excluded from the index. This results in a somewhat higher value than does the method for MLU computation, particularly in Brown's Stages I and II. Forms and construction in the transcript are scored and sorted into categories on a "Sequence of Language Acquisition" worksheet. Each is marked correct, incorrect, or absent in obligatory context. Forms and constructions are finally assigned to six categories relative to the level assigned the child by the word/morpheme index. Those present that are at or above the child's level are considered baseline structures. Those whose usage is below the assigned level are considered goals for remediation. Jay's baseline and goal worksheets are shown in Figure 3.

Jay's word/morpheme index is 3.68 by this analysis and is assigned to Level III. The forms and constructions that appear on his goal data worksheet are:

Pronouns:	*she**, *them**, *I, he, they, mine*
Plurals:	/s/*, /z/, /əz/*
Conjunctions:	*and**
Modals:	*hafta**, *will*
Particles:	*up, down*
Copula:	*is, 's, is are*
Auxiliary:	*is*
Third person singular:	/s/, /z/, *does*
Past tense:	regular, irregular

The items marked with an asterisk* do not appear in the transcript; the others appear but are used inconsistently. The LSAT contains no caveat on this score, but caution should be used in developing remedial procedures for structures that simply do not appear in the transcript. The transcript is, after all, only a sample. One would not necessarily expect everything the child knows to appear in it. This is particularly important considering that the recommended sample size is 100 utterances. Only with a larger sample taken in a variety of contexts, including attempts to elicit missing constructions, could the absence of a form be considered a definite problem.

GRAMMAR WRITING

In addition to comparing the LARSP, DSS, ASS, MLU, 14 morpheme, and LSAT methods of grammatical analysis, a generative grammar for the speech sample under investigation was written. The original purpose in writing the generative grammar was to compare the grammar, which was thought to represent the most complete form of analysis, with the other methods of analysis that were felt to be "shortcuts" in the sense that they classified sentences into predetermined categories. With an individual grammar it is possible to observe and describe the structures that actually appear in the speech sample and to devise a unique formalization for them. There are, however, problems inherent to the grammar writing process.

The first arises from the fact that we are dealing with a *sample* of the child's speech. This is related to what linguists call the competence/performance distinction. That is, we assume that a speaker has some implicit knowledge of the rules of the language (competence) that underlies the production of sentences. For a variety of reasons, this knowledge is not always applied perfectly in the act of talking (performance). Linguists have considered speech to be a somewhat unreliable indicator of knowledge of a language, since people make mistakes, get careless, and operate under certain memory and attention constraints when talking. A linguist would not want to conclude that a person does not "know" a rule simply because he or she does not use it in a short sample of speech or even because he or she occasionally uses it incorrectly.

In studying Jay's transcript, we are repeatedly faced with the problem of deciding whether he lacks particular rules of adult grammar simply because we do not see them used in this sample. We also face the problem of deciding how to treat variability in the rules Jay uses. In the early studies of child language, Brown (1973) and Cazden (1968) set the criterion for rule acquisition at 90% correct usage in obligatory contexts. In other words, only when a child used a grammatical form correctly in 90% of the situations in which adult grammar requires it, was the child given credit for having acquired the rule. But considering the competence/performance distinction especially in children just acquiring rules, it would not be surprising if factors such as memory and attention had a good deal of influence over whether or not rules in the process of being mastered were allowed to operate. If a rule appears to operate correctly some of the time, we might want to give the child credit for its productive use, since the child's grammar does in

Table 2. DSS analysis of transcript

Name: Jay   Recording Date: 3-9-78   Birth Date: ______

CA: 3;5   DSS: 4.20 (< 10th percentile)

	Transcript Number	Indefinite Pronoun	Personal Pronoun	Primary Verb	Secondary Verb	Negative	Conjunction	Interrogative Reversal	Wh-Q	Sentence Point	Total
		31	40	59	17	19	3	3	12	26	210
19	I gotta leave it up there.										
20	See?										
22	You can't put gas in there.										
23	No, watch.										
25	This is where the gas.										
26	Turn it this 'round.										
31	I don't know.										
32	It gets fire.										
*33	What happen?			—					2	0	2
37	Look at that hole.	1		1						1	3
39	We can get it out.	1	3	4						1	9
40	I got it.	1	1	—						0	2
42	Lookit.			1						1	2
43	I want some of those people.	3	1,3	1						1	9
47	What this say?	1		—				—	2	0	3
49	I can't do it.	1	1	4		4				1	11
51	I can't.		1	inc.		4				1	6
54	This say the barber shop.	1		—						0	1
55	This is the fire house?	1		1				↑		0	2
57	This is the fire thing?	1		1				↑		0	2
58	What's this?	1		1				1	2	1	6
60	What are this thing?	1		—				1	2	0	4
61	No, this is barber shop.	1		1						0	2
62	You gotta fit in here.		1	—	2					0	3

65	Let me get in there.		1	1	2					1	5
67	Me hurt my arm.		-,1	2						0	2
68	Danny give me it. (For "Danny gave it to me.")	1	1	—						0	2
71	There ain't no more.	-, 3		—		—				0	3
73	Turn it around!	1		1						1	3
75	This going up.	1		—						0	1
76	It's getting fire.	1		1						0	2
78	Where is them?		—	—				1	2	0	3
79	Oh, there's the fire.			1						1	2
80	See that fire hat?	1		inc.				inc.		1	2
81	It's a fire.	1		1						1	3
81A	See the fire?			inc.				inc.		1	1
84	These are the firemans.		3	2						0	5
85	It's a big man in there.	1		1						1	3
86	I'll get fire.		1	4						0	5
89	Here's the fireman.			1						1	2
90	He's trying to get him out.		2, 2	1	5					1	11
92	This is the elevator.	1		1						1	3
95A	Now her getting off the elevator.		—	—						0	0
96	Bring the other people.	3		1						1	5
97	That doesn't go.	1		6		7				1	15
103	No, her momma say, "No."		2	—						0	2
104	Then the fire would kill him.		2	6						1	9
105	You can jump.		1	4						1	6
108	Me wanna go outside.		—	1	2					0	3
108A	"Doggie, come up," and now, okay.			1			3			0	4
109	The fire comes up.			2						0	2
110	You gotta go to bed right now!		1	—	2					0	3
112	"('Cause) I don't want to."		1	4	inc.	4				1	10
113	This guy is.	1		inc.						1	2
114	He hurt himself.		2, 5	1						1	9
116	What that fire engine doing up on the roof?	1		inc.-				—	2	0	3
117	They wanna sleep together.		3	1	2					1	7
118	I wanna get out now.		1	1	2					1	5

*The last 50 S-V utterances of sample used for DSS (Lee, 1974, p. 67).

A	Unanalysed			Problematic	
	1 Unintelligible 10	2 Symbolic Noise	3 Deviant	1 Incomplete 4	2 Ambiguous 1

B	Responses		Repetitions	Normal Response						Abnormal		Problems
				Elliptical Major				Full Major	Minor	Structural	Ø	
Stimulus Type		Totals		1	2	3	4					
121	Questions	87	3	16	7	4		21	35	2	21	2
103	Others	16	4	1	1			3	5	1	1	
C	Spontaneous	70		8	Others 62							

Stage	Sentence Type						
Stage I (0;9–1;6)	Minor	Social	Stereotypes	Problems			
	Major	Sentence Structure					
	Excl.	Comm.	Quest.	Statement			
		"V"	"Q" 6	"V" 2	"N" 3	Other 4	Problems

Stage	Excl.	Comm.	Quest.	Conn.	Clause	Phrase	Word
Stage II (1;6–2;0)		Vx 1	Qx 2		SV 10, VC/O 2, SC/O 8, AX 2, Neg X, Other 6	DN 24, VV, Adj N 8, V part 9, NN, Int X 3, PrN 4, Other 3	-ing 6, pl 5, -ed 3
Stage III (2;0–2;6)		VXY 5, *let XY* 1, *do XY*	4 QXY, VS 3		X+S:NP 3, X+V:VP 2; SVC/O 21, VC/OA 3, SVA 6, VO_dO_i, Neg *XY* 1, Other	X+C/O:NP 11, X+A:AP; D Adj N 6, Cop 5, Adj Adj N 1, Aux 24, Pr DN 2, Pron 52, N Adj N, Other 4	-en 1, 3s 4, gen 0
Stage IV (2;6–3;0)		+S	QVS, QXYZ		XY+S:NP 1, XY+V:VP 3; SVC/OA 4, AAXY 1, SVO_dO_i 1, Other	XY+C/O:NP 14, XY+A:AP 6; N Pr NP, Neg V 8, Pr D Adj N, Neg X, cX, 2 Aux, XcX 1, Other 3	n't 12, 'cop 5, 'aux 3
Stage V (3;0–3;6)	*how*, *what*		tag	*and*, c, s, Other 6	Coord. 1, 1+; Subord. 1, 1+; Clause: S; Clause: C/O; Comparative	Postmod. 1 clause, 1+; Postmod. 1+ phrase	-est 0, -er 0, -ly 0

Stage VI (3;6–4;6)	(+)			(−)		
	NP	*VP*	*Clause*	*NP*	*VP*	*Clause*
	Initiator, Coord	Complex	Passive, Complement	Pron 7, Det 2, Adj Seq, N irreg 1	Modal 1, Tense 5, V irreg	Concord 2, A position, W order 1
	Other			Other Cop 13 Aux 2		

Stage VII (4;6+)	*Discourse*		*Syntactic Comprehension*
	A Connectivity	*it*	
	Comment Clause	*there*	*Style*
	Emphatic Order	Other	

Total No. Sentences	153	Mean No. Sentences Per Turn	1.22	Mean Sentence Length	2.82

Figure 2. LARSP Profile chart: Developmental stages. (©D. Crystal, P. Fletcher, and M. Garman, 1975 University of Reading, reprinted by permission.)

Language Sampling, Analysis, and Training: Baseline Analysis
D. Tyack and R. Gottsleben

Child *Jay* Age *3;5* Sex (M) F Sample Date ______

Referral Source ______ Clinician ______ Level: *III*

Reasons for Referral:

Background Information:

Data for items A through F on this form are obtained from the Sequence of Language Acquisition form. With the child's Level as a reference point, list below forms and constructions mastered; list on the reverse side, forms and constructions which appear inconsistently or not at all in his language sample. In planning for training on Negatives, Questions, and Complex Sentences, refer directly to the SLA form since these categories are not summarized on this form.

BASELINE DATA

A. Forms and constructions mastered* *at and below* assigned level.

Forms:

Pronouns
II me
my
it
III you
Prep
II in
on
III with
to

Demo:
I that
II this
III these
Locatives:
I here, there
Articles
II a, the

Modals
I wanna
II gonna
Pres progressive
II -ing

Constructions
I N, Mod+N, Quant+N
Poss+N, V+N, N+V
N+Ø cop + N/adj.
II V+Mod+N
N+V+N
III V+N+N, M+V+N
N+V+N+N

B. Forms and constructions mastered* *above* assigned level:

Forms:

Pronouns:
IV him
we
V her (poss.)
Prep
IV up
V down, off, of, at

Demo:
IV those
Modals
IV can
V can't
don't
gotta
won't

Constructions:
IV N+M+V
N+M+V+N(+N)

C. Unclassifiable forms and constructions:

right over there
my too little
the other ( ) over there
This is where the gas...
down the bathroom
right here
get burned

*Mastery is defined as correct occurrence of the structure 90% or more in obligatory contexts.

Figure 3. Language Sampling, Analysis, and Training: Baseline analyses and goal. (Reproduced by special permission from Language Sampling, Analysis and Training by Dorothy Tyack and Robert Gottsleben, ©Copyright 1974, published by Consulting Psychologists Press, Inc.

GOAL DATA

D. Forms and constructions *at or below* the assigned level which *do not appear:*

Forms:

Pronouns:	Modals	Constructions
III she, them	III hafta	I Adj. + N
Plurals:	Particles	V
II -s, -z	I up, down	
III -əz		
Conjunctions		
III and		

E. Forms and constructions *at or below* assigned level which appear *inconsistently* (i.e., less than 90% in obligatory contexts). Show these as fractions with no. of correct responses over no. of obligatory contexts.

Forms:

Pronouns:	Capula	Constructions
I I	III is, 's is aux	III N + is + N/adj.

F. Forms and constructions *above* the assigned level which appear inconsistently:

Forms:

Pronouns:	Copula	Constructions
IV he, they	IV are	
V mine	3rd pres	
Modals	IV -s, -z, does	
IV will	Past	
	V /d/, irreg.	

Other factors relevant to training program:

Figure 3. *(continued)*

fact sometimes generate well-formed sentences by means of this rule. We could then hypothesize that correct sentences were generated by a grammatical rule that is sometimes prevented from operating by performance constraints. If the rule is a fairly recent acquisition, we might conjecture that it would require extra attention, focusing, or planning and would therefore be more susceptible to violation than stable rules. Such performance factors might account for some of the variability with which the rule is used.

Whether or not this speculation as to the reason for variable application of grammatical rules is correct, the fact that the transcript reveals several cases of variable use requires a grammar to describe this variation in some way. It would not be satisfactory merely to accept the criterion of 90% correct usage and say that Jay does not "have," for example, a contractible copula. He clearly *has* it, since he uses it about 50% of the time, and in writing a grammar we must assume that it is generated in these instances by a rule. We want the grammar to provide a mechanism for generating variable forms, although we may set aside for the moment the question of why they are used only variably.

For these reasons, we have made the decision to abandon the traditional criterion for acquisition. In cases where there is greater than 90% but less than 100% correct usage, we will revert to the usual procedure and consider these forms stable acquisitions, rather than including them among the variable rules. (We have only one instance of less than 100% but greater than 90% correct usage—the articles *a* and *the* in obligatory contexts.) For those forms or constructions used in 50%–90% of the obligatory contexts, we will hypothesize the existence of a grammatical rule that is applied variably because of unspecified performance constraints. The lower limit is arbitrary. In Jay's sample all the forms that appeared were used in at least 50% of their obligatory contexts. Also, we would not want to attribute knowledge of a rule to the child if the rule were applied only once. We would want to see some repeated use in a variety of lexical and situational contexts in order to hypothesize that the rule is in fact productive.

Another problem with grammar-writing involves the assumption of the model of adult grammar. This assumption is made because the adult grammar is the language children are learning. To write a grammar, we formalize the rules we see operating, using the same conventions used to formulate rules for adult grammar, and note similarities and departures when they occur. There are two dangers in this approach, however. The first is that the formal characterization of many aspects of adult grammar is still a matter of debate among linguists. There is no complete adult grammar that is universally accepted to which we can refer. The model used here has been a relatively standard transformational approach (Akmajian and Heny, 1975) that is generally accepted among linguists, although points of disagreement still exist in many of its details. The model proposes that there are a set of phrase structure rules that specify the constituents of base sentences and show the hierarchical order and relations among these constituents. Transformations are hypothesized to act on these base sentences to produce derived structures, or variants of deep structures. These transformations may reorder elements ("I called up Jan"→"I called Jan up"), insert elements ("Three kids are on tape"→"There are three kids on tape"), or delete elements ("Give it *to* me"→"Give me it"), and copy elements into another part of the sentence ("She doesn't like yogurt"→ "She doesn't like yogurt, *does* she?"). This much of the model is generally accepted, but when it comes to formalizing some of the phrase structure and transformational rules, disagreements occur. We have simply accepted the Akmajian and Heny formulations as representative of a fairly conservative linguistic position. However, we must bear in mind that these rules, to which we are comparing those we can write for children, are not "proven" in any sense. There is always a risk that the model to which the child's grammar is being compared is in error.

A second danger in comparing the child's grammar to the adult's lies in the possibility that the child does not acquire adult grammar directly during the language-learning period. It is possible that children construct a preliminary set of rules that will later be reanalyzed into the adult system. Ingram (1975) suggests, for example, that the preoperational child may develop only a phrase structure grammar that generates complex sentences by juxtaposition of simple sentences, not by transformational rules. The phrase structure grammar is not reorganized to include transformations, according to Ingram, until the child achieves concrete operations. The grammar written for Jay ignores the possibility of this kind of restructuring and assumes that adult grammar is a valid model for describing the child's system. However, we should be aware that this assumption may be incorrect.

Mechanics of Writing a Grammar

In order to write a grammar, we must first choose sentences to include in it. We decided to use only those that contained both a noun phrase and a verb phrase (unless the sentence was a command), since this is the standard definition of a sentence. We did not want to be in the position of saying that the child had "omitted" a complete subject or predicate because these "omissions" are often the correct form of answering questions in conversation. To avoid penalizing Jay for answering questions in the pragmatically appropriate way, we simply excluded those utterances that consisted of either a noun phrase or verb phrase alone.

Next we assigned each word in the sentence to one of the following categories:

noun (N)
personal pronoun (pron)
verb (V)
adjective (adj)
demonstrative pronoun (demo pron)
preposition (prep)
adverb (adv)
determiner (det)

Under the verb category there were certain subclassifications:

auxiliaries (aux): modals (M), catenatives (cat)
copula (cop): *be* and its forms

As the words were labeled, the following sentence constituents were also identified:

sentence (S)
noun phrase (NP)
verb phrase (VP)
auxiliary (aux)

The NP, VP, and aux of each sentence were then listed. For example, the sentence "We can get the firetruck" would be described as follows:

NP→pron
aux→M
VP→V det N
(The symbol→is read: "is expanded as")

After the constituents of each sentence had been listed, the various expansions of NP, aux, and VP were collapsed into a set of phrase structure rules. When the phrase structure rules had been written, another pass was made through the transcript to look for transformations. This was done by simply identifying sentences that did not exhibit the standard NP-aux-VP form. In each case, the base structure of these sentences was identified and written out, and the type of transformation that appeared to generate the surface sentence was noted. Negative sentences and questions were considered to include obligatory transformations to place the negative and question elements. For example, the sentence "You can't put gas in there" would be analyzed as follows:

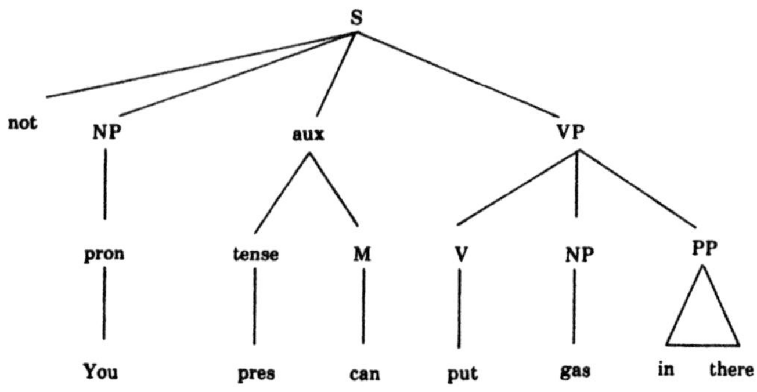

(Read: apply negative insertion and contraction transformations)

→negative insert,
contraction

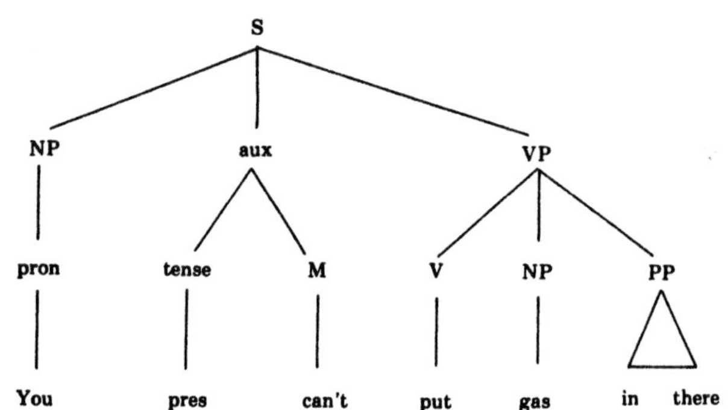

Each transformed, or nonkernal, sentence was analyzed to discover whether or not it fit the adult model. When a sentence did not, an attempt was made to write a new rule that could systematically generate utterances like the ones present in the transcript.

The following symbols were used in writing the phrase structure rules:

{ } rows within the braces are mutually exclusive. If one row is chosen, no other can be.
( ) what is inside the parentheses is optional; i.e., it may or may not be chosen.
({ }) either one row within the braces or nothing may be chosen.
< >% We have borrowed Labov's (in Wolfram and Fasold, 1974) angle-brace notation to indicate variable usage of a constituent, and have noted its percentage of occurrence.

Elements not enclosed in braces or parentheses are obligatory.

The following are the phrase structure (PS) rules for Jay's grammar:

$$S \rightarrow \left(\begin{Bmatrix} Q \\ \text{not} \end{Bmatrix}\right) NP\ aux\ VP$$

$$NP \rightarrow (det)\ (adj)\ N\ (pp)$$

$$aux \rightarrow tense\ \left(\begin{Bmatrix} M \\ cat_1 \\ \langle be \rangle_{57\%} \begin{Bmatrix} ing \\ cat_2 \end{Bmatrix} \end{Bmatrix}\right)$$

$$VP \rightarrow \begin{Bmatrix} \langle cop \rangle_{50\%}\ NP \\ \text{-cop}\ \begin{Bmatrix} adj \\ adv \end{Bmatrix} \\ V\ (NP)\ \begin{Bmatrix} (NP) \\ (pp)\ (adv)\ (adv) \end{Bmatrix} \end{Bmatrix}$$

$$det \rightarrow \begin{Bmatrix} \text{possessive pron} \\ \text{article} \\ \text{quantifier} \\ \text{demo adj} \end{Bmatrix}$$

$$adj \rightarrow (adv)\ adj$$

$$N \rightarrow \begin{Bmatrix} \text{demo pron} \\ \text{pron} \\ \text{noun} \end{Bmatrix}$$

$$tense \rightarrow \begin{Bmatrix} \text{present} \\ \langle \text{past} \rangle_{60\%} \end{Bmatrix}$$

$$M \rightarrow \begin{Bmatrix} \text{can} \\ \text{will} \end{Bmatrix}$$

$$cat_1 \rightarrow \begin{Bmatrix} \text{gotta} \\ \text{wanna} \\ \text{lemme} \end{Bmatrix}$$

$$cat_2 \rightarrow \begin{Bmatrix} \text{gonna} \\ \text{trynta} \end{Bmatrix}$$

$$cop \rightarrow \text{be}$$

$$pp \rightarrow \text{preposition NP}$$

Analyzing the Phrase Structure Rules

Our analysis reveals that it is possible to write a phrase structure grammar for Jay that closely resembles the phrase structure grammar we would write for an adult. At the sentence level, Jay's grammar contains at least three sentence types: statements, negative statements, and questions. Adults may have a greater variety of underlying sentence types in their repertoire, and indeed Jay may have more than those we find in this sample. But he is at least able to produce sentences that negate and question.

Jay's NP elaborations are similar in form to those of adults. The NP contains optional determiner and adjective elements that always occur before the noun and an optional prepositional phrase that follows it. An adult grammar would contain a greater variety of NP elaboration, including embedded sentences. We will consider the matter of embedding more fully in the analysis of the auxiliary system. As we will state many times in this section, we cannot be sure that Jay cannot embed simply because he does not in this sample. We do have some evidence for not giving him credit for complex sentences, however, which we will explore in the next section.

In discussing NP elaboration, we are being somewhat less complete and explicit than we would be in the ASS procedure. We have not specified the inclusion of particular prepositions, for instance. We have merely noted the appearance of *classes* of words. A complete grammar would include lexical (word) insertion rules for each of the grammatical classes. We have not gone this far, except in cases where errors of lexical insertion are committed (in the case of pronouns), or where a very limited number of words is involved (catenatives). By looking at lexical insertion rules for only a few word classes, we do lose some information.

The auxiliary component of English is one constituent of adult grammar that is acquired over the course of several stages of language development. We would expect, then, to see some variation from adult grammar in Jay's auxiliary system. The auxiliary PS rule for adult grammar is usually written as follows:

aux → tense {(M) (have -en) (be -ing)}

indicating an obligatory tense element (expanded as *past* or *present*) that may be followed by a modal (*can, will, must,* or *may*), *have* and its accompanying perfective affix (*-en*), and *be* with the progressive affix (*-ing*). In the generative model, these affixes are placed on the verb following each auxiliary element by a transformation called "affix hopping." Since the last three elements are in parentheses, one, two, all, or none of them may be chosen, but those used will be placed in the order specified in the rule. Therefore, sentences like the following are possible in adult grammar:

She pres will have en be ing live here for a year → (affix hopping)
She will have been living here for a year.

He past have en be ing wash dishes → (affix hopping)
He had been washing dishes.

It past may be ing rain → (affix hopping)
It might be raining.

They past get a new car → (affix hopping)
They got a new car.

The rule for Jay's auxiliary system is quite different, however. The first obvious difference is the absence of *have* and its perfective affix. There is no evidence of this form anywhere in the transcript, although, of course, we cannot be sure it does not exist in Jay's grammar. There are obligatory contexts for auxiliary *have,* however, in which it never appears. Nor does the catenative *hafta* show up. These facts lend some credence to the assertion that *have -en* is absent from the system.

The second major difference between Jay's rule and the traditional adult formulation lies in the inclusion of catenatives in the auxiliary. Most researchers in child language (Brown, 1973) have considered catenatives to be unanalyzed wholes rather than combinations of affixed verb and infinitives (e.g., gonna=going to). To consider the catenatives as main verbs requires us to analyze the verb phrases that follow them as embedded sentences, because the definition of a simple sentence requires that it takes only one main verb. Since there is no evidence of any other form of complex sentence in Jay's sample if we exclude sentences containing catenatives, and since the catenatives appear to function more like modals than like main verbs, we have decided to include them within the auxiliary.

We have subcategorized the catenatives into two groups. The first set includes *gotta, wanna,* and *lemme.* Although *lemme* is not usually considered a catenative, we have placed it in this group because it appears to function as an unanalyzed whole and because to consider it a main verb would require us, again, to give credit for complex object complements that is not justified by other evidence in the transcript. The words in this group are similar in that they appear to contain no affix. They are simply "stuck in," as modals are, before main verbs. They have no effect on the form of the following verb. They are also never preceded by another aux constituent. The second set of catenatives, *gonna* and *trynta,* shows evidence of being analyzed by the child as containing an affix *-ing.* This evidence lies in the fact that a form of auxiliary *be* sometimes precedes these words, just as it sometimes precedes other progressive forms. This distinction between catenative groups reveals a relationship of possible interest in auxiliary development. It appears that the forms containing implicit *-ing* begin to be analyzed before *gotta,* which contains implicit *-en* and requires a preceding *have.* We have pointed out that the auxiliary *be* appears frequently, although variably, in the transcript, while the auxiliary *have* does not appear at all. There may be a relationship between the child's analysis of catenative forms and the degree to which he controls the other auxiliaries that accompany them. This implies that the transition from catenatives to analyzed forms may take place individually, in accordance with relations to other aspects of the auxiliary system, rather than as a class. This would not be surprising because many other aspects of child grammar develop in this way (Slobin, 1973).

Note that in the LSAT, Jay is given credit for complex sentences containing *trying to,* simply because the catenative *trynta* does not appear in their list. It is clear from the transcript, however, that *trynta* only appears as an incompletely analyzed form, that sentences containing it parallel other catenative-containing sentences, and that there are no other instances of complement-taking verbs in the sample. Other differences between Jay's auxiliary system and that of adults are the absence of the modals *may* and *must* and the variable use of the auxiliary *be* with progressive verbs and catenatives.

There is some justification for postulating a *tense* element in Jay's auxiliary system. He marks verbs for *past* inconsistently (67% of the irregular past forms are marked in obligatory context, as are 50% of the regular verbs). Since there is some indication of this distinction between tenses, we hypothesize that Jay's grammar contains a *tense* element and that the *past* markers are used variably.

Expansion of the verb phrase for verbs other than the copula *be* is again very similar to the grammar we would write for adults, and as we saw in the noun phrase, the main difference is the absence of embedded sentences. Jay can string two NPs together in an indirect object-direct object construction ("Give me it."). Prepositional phrases and adverbs appear in the VP, and it is possible to choose any, all, or none of the forms in a VP expansion.

Jay's use of the copula does depart from adult usage, however. When adult grammar requires a form of *be* before an adjective or adverb ("The girl *is* happy"; "Mommy *is* home"), Jay omits it consistently, at least in this sample. The situation is more complicated when an NP follows the copula, however. *Be* appears variably in this case. Length of sentence does not appear to be the determining factor, since the copula appears in some of the longer sentences and is absent in some of the shortest. In examining the transcript it becomes clear that there is a difference between its first and second halves in terms of *cop-NP* use. In the first 80 utterances scored, the copula was present in 12% of the obligatory contexts preceding an NP. In the second 80 utterances however, it was present in 75% of the *cop-NP* contexts. (There were approximately equal numbers of obligatory contexts in each half of the transcript.) One might hypothesize on the basis of these data that a practice or modeling factor is operating. Jay may be hearing the clinician's use of *cop-NP* constructions and modeling them in his own speech. We would expect something like this to happen with a form whose use is in transition, so that its appearance in input language might be particularly salient. It is interesting to note in this regard that Jay sometimes uses the wrong forms of the copula ("What are this thing?"; "Where is them?") in the second half of the sample. This fact, too, lends support to a "transitioning" hypothesis. As Jay attempts to expand the use of the copula in his speech, he is not yet in control of the forms required for particular linguistic contexts.

If this "transitioning" hypothesis is correct, it indicates that Jay is highly stimulable for the *cop-NP* construction. The LSAT suggests that this form be taught as part of a remedial program. But since Jay's usage implies that the copula (at least in the NP context) is highly stimulable, a wiser approach might simply be to model *cop-NP* constructions for the child and to expand them for him when they appear incomplete in his speech. When the NP becomes stable following the copula, a similar approach could be used with *cop* $\left\{ \begin{smallmatrix} \text{adj} \\ \text{adv} \end{smallmatrix} \right\}$. Structured remedial work can be reserved for constructions that show less spontaneous stimulability (pronouns, perhaps). Here it seems clear that a detailed analysis, including a search for constraints governing use of variable constructions in the child's speech, yields information with important remedial implications that would be overlooked by other analysis tools.

The next PS rule in the grammar involves the expansion of the element *determiner.* Here we note at least two major departures from adult grammar. We would expect to see a possessive form for nouns (NPs) in this category. Although Jay uses possessive pronouns, the possessive morpheme is never attached to nouns in this sample. Adult rules for the determiner might also include more combinations of elements, for example:

det → (art.) (ordinal no.) (cardinal no.) (adj)
the first three red ones . . .

But Jay only uses combinations of article and adjective ("a big man").

The adjective component in Jay's grammar reveals that he can optionally modify an adjective with an adverb ("That how many"). This is also common in adult usage.

The forms that can function as pronouns in Jay's grammar encompass those that function similarly in adult grammar. However, his lexical insertion rules for this category depart somewhat from those of adults. Standard English rules require that pronouns [+subjective] *(I, we, he, she, it, you, they)* be placed in subject position, while those marked [−subjective], or perhaps [+objective] *(me, him, them, her),* must be used as objects of verbs and prepositions. All Jay's errors with pronouns involve using a [−subjective] pronoun in subject position. This substitution is not consistent, however (22% me/I; 100% her/she; 50% them/they). Examination of the transcript reveals no overriding regularity that governs these substitutions. We might formalize this fact in this way:

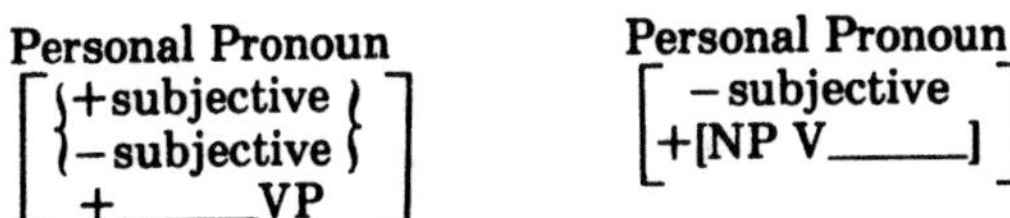

A subject *or* object pronoun may occur in subject position, while only an object pronoun can occur in object position. Although the grammar is not able to specify the context in which the object/subject substitution takes place, it does point out the systematic nature of Jay's pronominal errors.

The prepositional phrase in Jay's system has the same form as it does for adults, although the range of prepositions that appear in the sample is somewhat limited. As pointed out above, this grammar does not distinguish among the prepositions or score the ones Jay uses for order of acquisition. We merely give him credit for controlling this class of words.

The PS rules, then, have revealed a number of facts that were not evident from our other forms of analysis. First of all, they point out a lack of embedding, or complex sentence formation, in the elaboration of either noun or verb phrases. Jay's use of the copula is variable, with certain constraints. It never appears before an adjective or adverb alone. Its appearance before an NP increases in frequency in the second half of the transcript. We take this to indicate that Jay is modeling the clinician's use of copulas. Jay's errors in the use of personal pronouns consist only of substitutions of object for subject forms in subject position. His use of the auxiliary *be* with present progressive forms is variable (57%), although the *-ing* is realized in all cases. Jay's grammar appears to contain a tense element. The *past* aspect of tense is realized variably, however. Catenatives *(gonna, gotta, trynta,* and *lemme)* seem to function more like auxiliaries than main verbs, since there is no evidence in the transcript of any other main verbs that can take object complements to form complex sentences. However, there do seem to be subclasses within the catenatives. *Gonna* and *trynta* show evidence of being analyzed as containing an *-ing* affix since they are sometimes preceded by *be. Gotta, wanna,* and *lemme* show no such evidence.

Transformational Rules

In accordance with the decision to write a generative grammar for Jay's speech sample, we have made use of the notion of transformational rules. These rules add, delete, reorder, or copy elements in base sentences to produce stylistic variations in surface utterances. Any utterance that does not exhibit the kernal NP-aux-VP form is hypothesized to be the result of one or more transformations performed on an underlying sentence.

The use of transformational rules in this sample is not meant to imply that these rules are considered "psychologically real" for the child. We have made no attempt whatsoever to address the question of how the grammar actually operates. Our purpose is only to *describe* a child's speech by means of the same conventions that have proved useful in describing the language of adults. To do so, we have taken a rather conservative generative model of adult grammar and simply asked, "Could these same hypothetical rules be used to describe the sentences seen in this transcript?" The intent of this grammar is to describe the child's system in as much detail as possible, and to compare it to the language of adults. No attempt has been made to explain the actual mechanisms by which the child's sentences are generated.

One example of a transformational rule that can be applied successfully both to the adult's and to Jay's grammar is called *reflexivization.* It has been formalized in the following way (Akmajian and Heny, 1975):

Reflexivization (obligatory)
SD: NP-aux-V-X-NP
     1   2   3   4   5
SC: 1   2   3   4   5   [+reflexive] Condition: 1=5

The formalization can be read as follows: SD (structural description) describes what we assume to be the underlying form of the sentence. In this case, it contains the familiar constituents noun phrase, auxiliary, verb, and an x that represents "anything or nothing." In other words, what comes between the main verb and the NP to be reflexivized is irrelevant to the reflexivization rule. The condition on the transformation states that element 1 must refer to the same person or thing as does element 5. The fact that the rule is obligatory tells us that when the structural description, including the condition 1=5, is met, the transformation must operate to produce the given SC (structural change). It changes element 5 to a reflexivized form. Since the only reflexivized forms in English are pronouns, the rule implies pronominalization. For the sentence from Jay's transcript "He hurt himself," we postulate the underlying structure

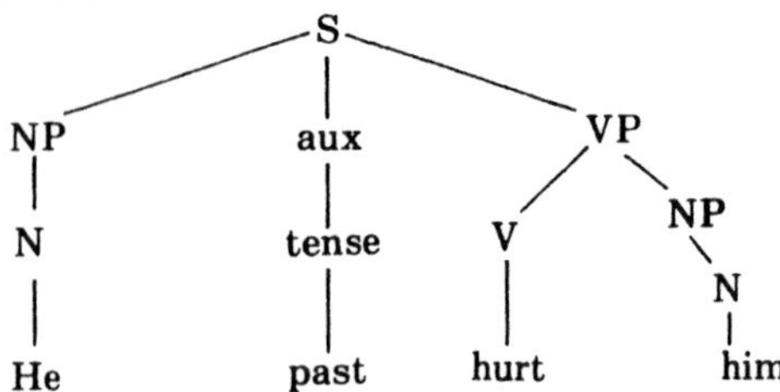

which is transformed by reflexivization to "He hurt himself." This rule can be said to operate for Jay as it does in adult grammar.

There is similar evidence for several other transformations that appear to function in this transcript as they do in adult speech. These include the placement of the negative element, the insertion of *there,* the placement of indirect objects, the formation of imperative sentences, and the contraction of negatives and verbs. Some of these appear only once or twice, so that it is difficult to know whether they function as rules or can only be used in a few memorized contexts. The "affix-hopping" transformation operates as it does in adult grammar only for those auxiliaries that have been fully analyzed by the child's system. The *-en* affix is never placed correctly, and past affixes are used inconsistently. The affix *-ing* is placed correctly in all contexts, even when the required form of *be* does not appear.

There are at least three contexts in which Jay's grammar cannot be described by the same transformation that applies to the adult system. The first involves number agreement, which in adults, chooses verb forms that agree with subjects in person and number. In Jay's sample, however, we sometimes find incorrect forms in these slots, for example, "Where is them?". Since there are instances of number agreement in the transcript both with forms of *be* and third person singular, we can conjecture that Jay does apply a number agreement transformation, but again, uses it variably, perhaps as a result of performance constraints. (The 14 morpheme analysis also deals in part with this issue, in looking at third person singular forms. It is a more limited analysis, however, because it only looks at a particular set of instances of agreement and not at the various forms of *be.* In doing the 14 morpheme analysis, we count only the correct appearance of *be* and do not distinguish between absent and incorrect forms.) The variability of this rule in Jay's grammar might be interpreted either to mean that the rule is not stable and so is not always applied, or that the particular forms to be used in agreement have not been fully analyzed. We cannot really choose an interpretation on the basis of this sample, but the existence of the general agreement rule and its variability is of interest in planning a remedial program.

There are two other transformations that appear to operate as unstable acquisitions in the sample. They are the Wh-question and "do-support" transformations. Yes/no questions appear to be marked only by rising intonation, although we cannot be sure Jay never inverts subject and auxiliary to form the adult yes/no question. Jay is sometimes able to form Wh-questions but it is interesting to note that in three of the six instances of these questions, something else "goes." "Where is them?" and "What are this thing?" involve incorrect number agreement. "What happen?" shows absence of past tense affix. In other Wh-questions, the auxiliary or copula is simply omitted, although there are two instances of correct inversion.

Jay's use of the "do-support" transformation is related to his use of questions. "Do-support" provides for *do* to be inserted when an affix is "stranded" without an immediately following verb by the insertion of *not* or the formation of a question. Although its description is not a matter of complete agreement among linguists, it can be tentatively formalized as follows:

SD:	x	tense	
	1	2	
SC:	1 do #	2	Conditions: x is not M or V

In other words, "do-support" will only operate when *tense* is not adjoined to a verb. This situation occurs after a negative insertion or question transformation has operated. For example:

He pres go→(neg insertion) He pres not go
(affix hopping)→He pres not go (The transformation is blocked because no V follows *tense.*) insert *do*
(affix hopping)→He does not go.

Jay inserts *do* correctly in all negative sentences that require it. In questions requiring *do,* he consistently omits it.

It appears from this analysis that in forming questions, Jay sometimes abandons rules that are at least somewhat stable when he forms statements. The question transformation itself does not appear to be completely formulated in Jay's system, and its application seems to have the effect of disrupting the application of other rules that can apply in conjunction with it; most notably number agreement, "affix-hopping," and "do-support." In the case of "do-support" there is evidence that it is violated only in the context of questions and is relatively stable in negative statements.

All this leads to a rather simple conclusion: Jay has trouble forming Wh-questions. Although this point would probably be clear from the other forms of analysis as well, the examination of transformations does reveal that not only is Wh-question-formation itself a problem, but it also appears to affect the application of other rules that may accompany it. We might go so far as to say the application of the question transformation decreases the probability of correct application of number agreement, "affix-hopping," and "do-support."

Our analysis of Jay's use of transformations reveals that those that are most unstable are those that concern auxiliaries and their effects on main verbs. This corroborates our analysis of Jay's PS grammar in that there, too, the greatest departures from the adult system were seen in the auxiliary component. This should not come as any surprise since we know from research in child language that the English auxiliary system takes a long period of time to develop.

In general terms, then, the grammar we have written for Jay points out the same areas of difficulty as do some of the other analyses. But the grammar also gives information about constraints on particular constructions, environments in which constructions are more or less likely to occur, and the interaction of some linguistic processes with others. The ASS and the LSAT come closest to the grammar in providing descriptive information about the structures that turn out to be most important for making remedial decisions for Jay. When we compare the level of detail afforded by the grammar with that of the other tools, the descriptive advantages of ASS and LSAT become clear. This high degree of descriptiveness is most useful in planning a remediation program. There may even be times when a clinician interested in prescribing remedial activities would write a partial grammar for those aspects of the system identified as problems by another analysis. This procedure could highlight such qualities as stimulability or influence of some structures on others, and might help determine the order of remedial targets.

COMPARING ACROSS ANALYSES

The purpose in comparing these structural analyses has not been to select the one best procedure for all children. The goal is rather to discover how the analyses differ in the detail of description they yield. For example, how sensitive is a given procedure to the development of the auxiliary verb system? What information does it provide about question formation? In addition to comparing descriptive power we will also examine the analyses in terms of mechanical efficiency, since efficiency, too, is an important consideration in clinical work.

One way to compare the measures is to examine Jay's performance on each of them. Figure 4 illustrates Jay's scores with reference to chronological age on four of the measures. Note that the LSAT and generative grammar analysis provide no metric for estimating age-equivalence. The 14 morpheme analysis has not been included in Figure 4.

The first measure, MLU, was plotted using the MLU-age linear prediction equation derived by Miller and Chapman (Chapter 2, this volume). Based on Jay's MLU of 3.06 morphemes, the equation would predict an age equivalent of 35 months. The vertical index for this measure represents ± one standard deviation plotted for the predicted age of 35 months, resulting in a range of normal variation between 33 and 46 months. Thus it is evident that Jay's MLU falls within normal limits, even though his age predicted from MLU is 6 months below his CA. The Assigning Structural Stage analysis was plotted against CA, and a similar picture resulted. Jay's grammatical system, as viewed through the ASS analysis, resulted in an Early Stage IV level of development. The major portion of grammatical structures centered at Early Stage IV, with expected variability below this stage, but only two grammatical structures present above it.

Finally, Figure 4 shows that Jay's performance on both DSS and LARSP falls outside the range of normal variability. The variability limits for DSS are interpolated from measures of standard deviation around DSS. Lee also provides percentile data for comparison. Jay's DSS of 4.20 is below the 10th percentile for his CA.

The LARSP is not a standardized procedure, as the DSS is, and therefore provides no statistical measure of variability. However, Crystal et al. (1976) note that "a spread of ± 6 months is quite tolerable within the notion of 'normal age range'" (p. 84). Thus, we have placed this "normal age range" between 35 and 47 months for the LARSP. We estimate Jay's level of development on the LARSP to be between Stages III–IV (about 2;6 years). No conventions are given for stage placement; thus, our overall stage assignment is only our "best guess." Jay's grammatical level of approximately 30 months is below LARSP's range of normal variability by 5 months.

To summarize the first comparison (Figure 4), age-equivalence data are lacking for two of the procedures (LSAT and generative grammar), and the others yield differing interpretations of Jay's language functioning. Both MLU and the ASS place Jay's productive language system within normal bounds, while the DSS and LARSP conclude that Jay's language is below the range of normal variability.

There are several reasons for this discrepancy. As Miller outlines the procedure for assigning overall stage in ASS, the stage of usual performance, or most frequent stage, should be accompanied by variation in constructions both above and below this level. Jay does use structures below his usual level, but we see very few instances of constructions above it. Miller's procedure instructs us to assign Jay's sample to this usual level of performance, and does not give us a method for taking the lack of higher level structures into account. Miller warns, however, that performance, such as Jay's, with little evidence of emerging complex structures should alert the clinician to the need for follow-up assessment. Miller's procedure, because it gives the child credit for the highest level structures in the transcript, can result in a somewhat liberal stage assignment, although the stage assignments for individual constructions may be conservative. This tendency in ASS stage assignment procedure to compensate for conservative placement of individual structures by a more generous standard for overall stage assignment may explain the discrepancy between the ASS results and the DSS. Comparing ASS to the LARSP reveals that both analyses paint a similar picture of Jay's performance. Structures appear below the most frequent stage, but few appear above it. The age range predicted for Jay's stage of usual performance on the LARSP, however, is lower than the age data for ASS. This fact may be the result of the lack of standardization for both ASS and LARSP. Each procedure is based on the authors' interpretation of studies of normal language development, which are usually derived from small longitudinal samples. Large-scale cross-sectional studies to validate stage placements and age-equivalents are needed to resolve these discrepancies.

There are, then, differences among the results of the various procedures. ASS places Jay around age level although it points out a need for follow-up assessment. LARSP and DSS find him significantly delayed.

COMPARING FEATURES OF ANALYSIS PROCEDURES

Table 3 displays a set of features by which the analysis procedures can be compared. We chose those that contribute either to clinical efficiency or to descrip-

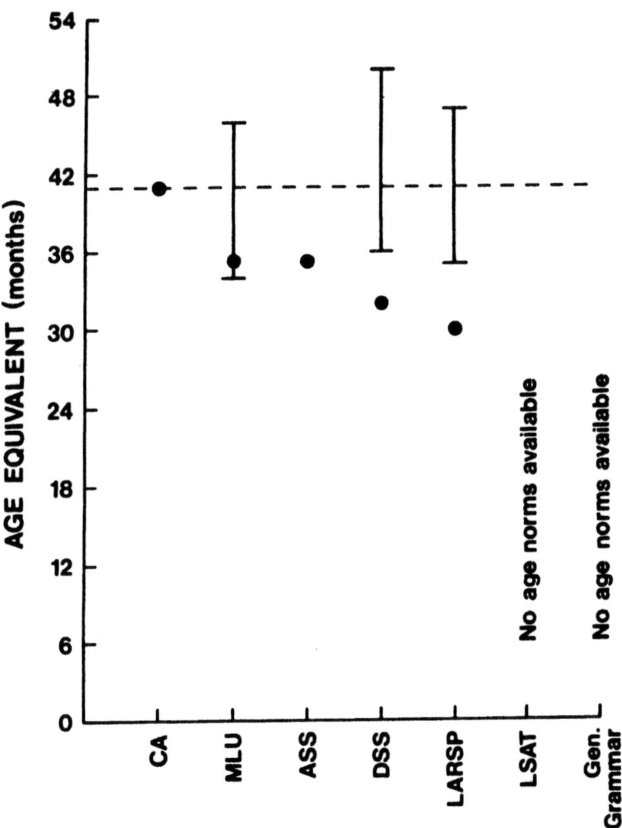

Figure 4. Summary scores for each analysis plotted relative to client's age of 41 months. Expected upper and lower limits of normal variability, plotted relative to age are represented by vertical bars. Each author's criterion for estimating normal variability was used. These are as follows:

MLU: −1 SD from 41 months (Miller, this volume, p. 26)
DSS: between upper and lower 10th percentile for 41 months (Lee, 1974, pp. 168–170)
LARSP: 6 months above and below client's age (Crystal, Fletcher, and Garman, 1976, p. 84)

tive power and scored each analysis as either containing (+) or lacking (−) each feature. We exclude the generative grammar from our discussion of mechanical properties, since we are only using it to compare details of specific grammatical information, not for its ease or efficiency of use.

The first category, prescribed analysis procedure, refers simply to whether or not there is a set of precise, detailed instructions available for doing the analysis, including worksheets for various sections. Such a set of instructions will make the procedure not only easier to use but also more reliable, since it will ensure that the analysis is done the same way for each child. The ASS, while containing a procedural outline, is less detailed in its mechanical aspects than the other procedures reviewed. This feature has been placed first on the list because we consider it to be of primary importance. In order to have confidence in an assessment tool we would want to be sure that each clinician performs the analysis in exactly the same way. Although the ASS is described in the manual we find the instructions to be less precise than those for other analyses. The set of categories to be analyzed is left up to the clinician's discretion, as is the choice of constructions within categories.

One might raise the objection that to prescribe the procedure precisely is to offer a "cookbook" approach that limits the clinician's ability to tailor the assessment to the needs of individual children. But because placement and treatment decisions may be made on the basis of the outcome of ASS, it is crucial to ensure that the procedure is reliable. Different clinicians should arrive at the same results when employing the analysis. A precise description of the format for choosing utterances to score, identifying constituents, and organizing them for stage assignment would not only decrease the time and effort required to complete the procedure, but would also increase its reliability in the hands of clinicians with varying levels of training and expertise. All the other procedures reviewed provide adequate procedural descriptions.

The next row in the table shows simply whether or not a worksheet summarizing the information in the procedure is provided. Such a worksheet makes analysis and stage determination quicker and easier, since the information is collapsed into a compact format. All of the procedures under investigation except the ASS provide this summary worksheet. Table 1 in this chapter presents one possible form for

Table 3. Features of language analysis procedures

Category	ASS: Structural	ASS: MLU	ASS: 14 Morpheme	DSS	LSAT	LARSP	Generative grammar
Prescribed analysis procedure	+	+	+	+	+	+	−
Summary worksheet	−	NA	−	+	+	+	−
Age equivalent	−	+	−	+	−	+	−
Developmental stage-assignment criteria							
Per constituent type	+	NA	+	+	+	+	−
Overall level	−	+	−	+	+	−	−
Measure of SD	−	+	−	+[a]	−	−	−
Informal measure of variability	+	NA	+	NA[a]	+	+	−
Does not require NP-VP for analysis	+	+	+	−	+	+	−
Linguistic comprehensiveness (i.e., broad range of constructions)	+	NA	−	−	+	+	+
Can incorporate new data	+	NA	−	−	−	−	NA
Specific grammatical categories							
Auxiliaries	+	−	+	+	+	+	+
Copula	+	−	+	+	+	+	+
Question forms	+	−	−	+	+	+	+
Determiners	+	−	+	+	+	+	+
Pronominalization	−	−	−	+	+	+	+
Verb inflections	+	−	+	+	+	+	+
Other morphological markers	−	−	+	−	+	+	+
Negation	+	−	−	+	+	+	+
Embedding	+	−	−	−	+	+	+
Adjectives	+	−	−	−	+	+	+
Required sample size for analysis		(15–30 minutes)		50 utterances	100 utterances	30 minutes	unspecified

+ = Feature present
− = Feature absent
NA = Not applicable
[a]Percentile norms included

a summary worksheet appropriate for a child at Jay's language level. Miller also gives a sample worksheet (see Table 9, Chapter 2), but no complete, all inclusive, standard form is given.

In the category labeled "age equivalent," we see that MLU, the DSS and the LARSP yield a direct age score. The DSS and MLU age scores are based on normative data. The ASS derives age from CA-MLU predictions and the LARSP draws age information from the developmental literature. Although the intent of the LSAT is to program for remediation, some measure of developmental equivalent score is essential in a language-analysis instrument. Without it the task of deciding whether or not the child really has a language problem that requires remediation becomes very difficult. After doing the LSAT we only discover which structures fall at or above the child's baseline and which fall below. We have no idea whether or not that baseline and variation around it correspond to age expectations. Some measure of developmental equivalent score, we believe, is an essential feature of a diagnostic tool.

Another feature of language assessment procedures identified as desirable is the assignment of various utterance constituents into stages of development. This is useful in identifying those structures, e.g., auxiliaries and question forms, in which the child may be delayed. By assigning a level or stage to each structure, the range of function across grammatical categories can be easily seen.

In addition, we have found it useful to assign a general stage of development to the child. Again, procedures for accomplishing this task should be explicitly specified by the author of the procedure. Procedures that provide explicit instructions for assigning overall stage of development are MLU, the DSS, and the LSAT. The LARSP and the ASS provide the raw data and guidelines for determining an overall stage of functioning, but lack an explicit convention for summarizing and interpreting the data by means of an overall stage assignment.

A measure of standard deviation is an extremely useful feature in a clinical tool, since it shows the range of difference from mean performance that can still be considered within limits of normal variability. Unfortunately, this measure has been very difficult to calculate for grammatical structures, because the data from which the developmental information is drawn has been gathered longitudinally from a small number of children. Only DSS and Miller and Chapman's data on MLU provide information on standard deviation. But MLU is, of course, only a general index of complexity in terms of utterance length and not a means of structural description.

Even an informal measure of variability is helpful. The LSAT and the LARSP each gives some indication of acceptable variation around the general developmental stage, but the measure of variability has not been standardized. The ASS proposes that one stage above and below MLU stage assignment represents normal variability.

Most speech samples will be drawn from conversation, and conversation characteristically contains incomplete sentences. An instrument that does not require a complete NP-VP sentence for analysis has the advantage of being able to use more of the sample in gathering information. All of these procedures except the DSS have this property.

The next category is labeled, rather vaguely, "linguistic comprehensiveness." By this we mean whether or not an analysis allows us to look at a broad spectrum of forms and constructions rather than limiting our view to a few selected constituents. The ASS analysis, the LARSP, and the LSAT provide the most comprehensive look at a language sample in terms of number of forms and constructions—with the exception, of course, of the individualized grammar.

Since all of these procedures rest upon a developmental model of language assessment, the capability for modification in light of new developmental research data is highly desirable. Norm-referenced procedures are not suited to this kind of modification. The ASS provides this flexibility. As new developmental information becomes available, clinicians can add it to the charts. Similarly, should placement of forms change with subsequent research, these data can replace present stage assignments. For example, information concerning personal pronoun development is not a part of the current child literature. As studies in this area emerge, the data can be incorporated into the charts. A second example is the case of Wh-question development. Stage placement of these constructions in the DSS is not congruent with current findings by Tyack and Ingram (1977) and by Chapman, Paul, and Wanska (in preparation). The ASS allows the clinician to make stage changes consistent with the most recent information available and thus keep the charts updated.

The rest of Table 3 can be seen as the set of elements that determines the larger category of linguistic comprehensiveness. A set of sentence constituents that we have found most useful in looking at language samples of children between Brown's stages II and V is specified. These structures are the ones in which developmental change is most likely to be seen. Again, the ASS, the LARSP, and the LSAT come closest to encompassing all the grammatical categories we would like to examine.

As Table 3 reveals, there are differences among the six standard analyses. These differences appear in both the mechanics and the content of the procedures. However, Table 3 is not meant to be used in a quantitative fashion. That is, it was *not* our intent that readers sum the pluses in each column and choose the procedure with the greatest number of features marked (+). This list of features is by no means complete, and the individual features may differ in importance. While mechanical efficiency is certainly a consideration in the clinic, a concern for linguistic comprehensiveness may often override it. Age-equivalence is certainly essential in diagnosis, but if we know a problem exists, remedial information, as offered by the LSAT, may be more useful than a description whose aim is age prediction. The clinician must determine the relative importance of each feature and choose the constellation of features that best suits each child in the caseload.

APPENDIX
Jay's Transcript

Name of child: Jay
DTU number:
Chronological age: 3;5
Date of evaluation: 3/9/78
Examiner: T. K.

Child MLU: 3.08
SD: 1.95
Number of utterances: 167
Sources of transcription: Audiotape

Examiner MLU: 5.68
SD: 3.08
Number of utterances: 224

Key:
T = Tom (examiner)
J = Jay
[ ] = Unintelligible utterance
[1 syllable] = Unintelligible, but number of syllables estimated from prosodic features
[MLU] = Morpheme count for child, based on Brown (1973).
* = Spontaneous utterances; nonresponses
(inc.) = Incomplete utterances, not counted in MLU. Morpheme count for all adult utterances based on adult morphological criteria.

Situation variables:
Time of day: 2:00 p.m.
Setting: WCMR
Materials used: Small toys, people, Playskool firehouse, etc.
Length of interaction: 30 minutes
Participants/Type of interaction: 1. T.K.—dyadic interaction
2.
3.
4.

Pragmatics		Speaker		Utterance Number	Dialogue	Morpheme Count		Syntax	Semantics
Child	Adult					Child	Adult		
		J		1.	*When are we gonna do that?	6			
			T		Do you know what that's called?		8		
		J		2.	What?	1			
			T		That's called a "tape recorder."		8		
		J			Oh.	1			
			T		Do you know what a tape recorder does?		10		
		J			Yeah.	1			
			T		Look at this.		3		
			T		I want to show you this.		6		
			T		Can I pin this on your shirt?		7		

Pragmatics		Speaker	Utterance Number	Dialogue	Morpheme Count		Syntax	Semantics
Child	Adult				Child	Adult		
		T		Would you like to wear this?		6		
		J		Yeah.	1			
		T		How about that!		3		
		T		Isn't that neat?		4		
		J	3.	*What are we gonna do with it?	7			
		T		Just leave it on your shirt.		6		
		T		I'll let you wear it while you're in here.		11		
		T		Would you like that?		6		
		J		Yeah.	1			
		T		Okay.		1		
		T		I want to show you a book here that I have.		11		
		T		You wanted to look at Paul's book and I want to show you this book.		17		
		T		This is a picture book.		5		
		T		Okay, I'd like you to tell me. . .		—		
		J	4.	*That a house.	3			
		T		What is it?		3		
		J	5.	A house.	2			
		T		Very good.		2		
		T		What's this?		3		
		J	6.	That a farm.	3			
		[Artic. test administered at this point]						
		T		You did a good job on that.		7		
		T		Now, I've got some toys we wanna play with.		12		
		J		Okay.	1			
		T		You stay here and I'll bring them over.		9		
		J		Okay.	1			
		T		Don't you want to wear this anymore?		9		
		J		No.	1			
		T		We'll just set that right on here.		8		
		T		Let me go get some of these toys.		9		
		T		I bet you've never seen one of these before; have you?		12		

J	7.	*That good.	2	
T		What is it?		3
T		What is that big thing?		5
J	8.	Car	1	
J	8a.	*Hey, the other [1] in over there.	7	
J	8b.	*Get the other [1] over there.	6	
T		Get the other what?		4
J	8c.	Other [1].	2	
T		I don't see it.		5
J	9.	*Yeah, right over there.	4	
T		Why don't you get it?		6
T		Can you reach your hand over there?		7
T		Mine are too big.		4
J	10.	I can't.	3	
T		You can't?		3
J	11.	No, my too little.	4	
T		That's a toilet.		4
T		Your hands are too little?		6
J		Yeah.	1	
J	12.	*See?	1	
T		What is that?		3
J	13.	A toilet.	2	
T		I don't think so.		5
T		I think it looks like a barber chair.		9
J	14.	It is a barber chair.	5	
T		Where do you suppose it goes?		7
T		Do you see a barber shop?		6
J	15.	*No, this doesn't work.	5[a]	
T		It doesn't work?		5
T		Is that supposed to open a door?		8
J		Yeah.	1	
T		You try it.		3
T		It doesn't work, does it?		8
J		Yeah. (laughter)	1	
T		What is that?		3
J	16.	A stop sign.	3	
T		You know what that says on there?		8
J	17.	What?	1	
T		That says, "Police Station."		5
J	18.	Oh, Police Station.	3	
J	19.	*I gotta leave it up there.	6	
T		You're gonna leave it up there?		9

continued

Pragmatics: Child	Pragmatics: Adult	Speaker	Utterance Number	Dialogue	Morpheme Count: Child	Morpheme Count: Adult	Syntax	Semantics
		J		Yeah.	1			
		J	20.	*See?	1			
		T		Why do you put it up there?		7		
		J		'Cause.	1			
		T		Can you see anything else?		6		
		J	21.	A gas.	2			
		T		A gas.		2		
		J	22.	*You can't put gas in there.	7			
		T		Why can't you put gas in there?		8		
		J		'Cause.	1			
		T		Can't you see an opening for gas?		9		
		J	23.	No, watch.	2			
		J	24.	*That a toy.	3			
		T		Well, how does the car go if it can't use gas?		13		
		J		'Cause.	1			
		J	25.	*This is where the gas.	5			
		T		This is where you gas?		5		
		J		Yes.	1			
		J		[ ].	—			
		T		Tell me again.		3		
		J	26.	*Turn it this 'round.	4			
		J	27.	*Another bath.	2			
		T		Another?		1		
		J	28.	Bathroom.	1			
		T		Another bathroom.		2		
		J		*What does this . . . (inc.)	—			
		T		What does this say?		5		
		T		This says "Firehouse."		5		
		J	29.	[sigh] Firehouse!	1			
		T		Where is the firehouse?		5		
		J	30.	Right here.	2			
		T		Jay . . . what happens when you turn this red handle?		10		
		J	31.	I don't know.	4			
		J	32.	It gets fire.	4			
		T		Why don't you turn it and see.		8		
		J	33.	*What happen?	2			
		T		I don't know.		4		
		J	34.	*That the fire.	3			
		T		That's the fire?		4		

		J			Yeah.		1	
			T			That's a siren.		4
			T			That's not a fire truck.		6
		J		35.	No, it a Volkswagen.		4	
			T			It's a what?		4
		J		36.	A Volkswagen.		2	
			T			A Volkswagen, right!		3
			T			I don't see the fire truck.		7
			T			Where is it?		3
		J		37.	*Look at that hole.		4	
			T			Look at that hole.		4
			T			Where does it go?		5
		J		38.	Down the bathroom.		3	
			T			Down the bathroom?		4
		J			Yeah.		1	
			T			There's somebody up in here.		7
		J		39.	*We can get it out.		5	
			T			You can get him out.		5
		J		40.	*I got it.		3	
			T			You got it?		3
		J			Yeah.		1	
			T			Good work.		2
		J		41.	*Here!		1	
			T			Thank you.		2
			T			Can he fit in your car?		6
		J			No!		1	
			T			That's too bad.		4
		J		42.	*Lookit.		1	
		J		43.	*I want some of those people.		6	
			T			You want some of those people.		6
			T			Who is that?		3
		J		44.	A girl.		2	
			T			A girl?		2
			T			And who is that?		4
		J		45.	A dog.		2	
					*I'm gonna be. . . (inc.)		—	
					*This can fit in my. . . (inc.)		—	
			T			Hey—do bears drive cars?		7
		J			Yeah.		1	
			T			They do?		2
			T			Have you ever seen a bear drive a car?		9
		J			Yeah.		1	
			T			You know what I'd like you to tell me?		10
		J		46.	What?		1	

continued

Pragmatics		Speaker	Utterance Number	Dialogue	Morpheme Count		Syntax	Semantics
Child	Adult				Child	Adult		
		T		Tell me about your monkey.		5		
		J	47.	*What this say?	3			
		T		That says, "Firehouse."		5		
		T		Can you tell me about the monkey at home?		9		
		T		What are you doing now?		6		
		J		[ ]	—			
		T		What's wrong?		3		
		J	48.	Gotta get this outta there.	5[b]			
		T		You gotta get this out of there?		7		
		J		Yeah.	1	1		
		T		Maybe this man can give you some help.		8		
		J	49.	*I can't do it.	5			
		T		Sure you can.		3		
		T		Watch this.		2		
		T		This man is gonna push it out the other way.		12		
		T		Here—use this to do it.		6		
		T		Whoops!		—		
		J	50.	Can't.	2			
		T		Almost.		1		
		J	51.	I can't.	3			
		T		You can't.		3		
		T		Watch this.		2		
		T		Push it back.		3		
		J	52.	*There!	1			
		J	53.	*What this say?	3			
		T		Barber shop.		2		
		J		*Oh!	—			
		J	54.	*This say the barber shop.	5			
		J	55.	*This is the fire house?	5			
		T		This is the fire house.		5		
		J	56.	*What this?	2			
		T		That's the mail house.		5		
		T		That's the post office.		5		
		J	57.	*This is the fire thing?	5			
		J	58.	*What's this?	3			
		T		That says "mail," and you know what?		8		
		J	59.	What?	1			

Speaker	No.	Utterance	J	T	Comments
T		That's a letter you can mail.		7	
J	60.	*What are this thing?	4		
T		That's a barber shop.		5	
J	61.	No, this is barber shop.	5		
T		Right!		1	
J	62.	*You gotta fit in here.	5		
T		That's a letter.		4	
T		Can you mail the letter?		5	
T		See the stamp?		3	
T		Where do you mail letters?		6	
J	63.	Right here.	2		
T		Okay, there's the mail box.		6	
J	64.	*Put this one in?	4		
T		Now, how do you get them out?		7	
J	65.	*Let me get in there.	5		
J	66.	*There.	1		
T		That's one.		3	
J	67.	*Me hurt my arm.	4		
T		Oh, let's see.		4	
T		What happened?		3	
J	68.	Danny give me it.	4		
T		How did Danny do that?		5	
J	69.	With *her* arm.	3		wrong use of pronoun gender
T		With her arm?		3	
J		Yeah.	1		
J	70.	*Two.	1		
T		You got two?		3	
J	71.	*There *ain't* no more.	4		scored as unanalyzed negation (III)
T		I think your car needs some more gas.		9	
T		What are you gonna do?		7	
J	72.	Gotta turn it around.	4		
T		Gotta turn it around.		5	
J	73.	Turn it around!	3		
T		I'll help you.		4	
T		Can you help me?		4	
J	74.	*There the stop sign.	4		
J	75.	*This going up.	4		
T		What's happening?		4	
J	76.	It's getting fire.	5		
T		Why?		1	
J		'Cause.	1		
T		Is the car broken?		5	
J		Yep.	1		
T		Who's gonna fix it?		7	
J	77.	The driver. . . the fire engines.	6		
T		The fire engines?		4	

continued

Pragmatics		Speaker	Utterance Number	Dialogue	Morpheme Count		Syntax	Semantics
Child	Adult				Child	Adult		
		J	78.	*Where is them?	3			
		T		Where is them?		3		
		J		Yeah.	1			
		T		I don't know.		4		
		T		Where are they?		3		
		J	79.	*Oh, there's the fire!	4			
		T		But where is it?		4		
		T		Where's the truck?		4		
		J	80.	*See that fire hat?	4			
		T		Uh-huh.		1		
		J	81.	*It's a fire.	4			
		T		But I don't see the fire truck.		8		
		J	81.a	*See the fire?	3			
		T		What are you trying to do?		7		
		J	82.	Get the guy out.	4			
		J	83.	*This guy.	2			
		J	84.	*These are the firemans.	5			
		J	85.	*It's a big man in there.	7			
		T		You know what?		3		
		T		Let's pretend.		3		
		T		Do you like to pretend?		5		
		J		Yeah.	1			
		T		Let's pretend that this lady is in the house, and this house is on fire.		16		
		T		Now, what are we gonna do?		8		
		J	86.	I'll get fire.	4			
		T		Okay, first we have to make a siren.		8		
		T		Now, what happens?		4		
		J	87.	Get burned.	3			
		T		Get burned?		3		
		J		Yeah.	1			
		T		You better get her out before she dies.		9		
		T		Send the fireman up.		5		
		T		Where's the fireman?		5		
		J	88.	I don't know.	4			
		J	89.	Here's the fireman!	4			
		T		Now, what's he doing?		6		
		J	90.	He's trying to get him out.	8			

Speaker	No.	Utterance	J	T
T		He's gonna get him out, good!		9
T		Hurry, because the flames are getting higher and higher!		13
T		Hurry!		1
T		We don't want her to burn.		7
T		Good work!		2
T		What does she say?		5
J	91.	Nothing.	1	
T		Doesn't she even say, "Thank you"?		8
J		Yeah.	1	
T		Boy, that fireman did a good job.		8
J		Yep.	1	
J		(unintell.)	—	
T		Tell me again.		3
J	91a.	Going up in the, [up in the, up in, up in the] [one syllable] get in bed.	9	
T		They're going up where?		6
J	91b.	Up in the [one syllable], get in bed.	7	
T		And they're gonna get in bed?		9
T		I bet they'd like to ride on the elevator.		10
J	92.	*This is the elevator.	4	
T		There's another one in the building.		7
J		Now. . .	1	
T		Now what happened?		4
J	93.	Get fire.	2	
T		How do they get down?		5
J	94.	I don't know.	4	
T		Did they like that?		4
J		Yeah.	1	
J	95.	*The girl happy.	3	
T		The girl happy.		3
T		That's great.		3
T		The dog wants to go.		6
T		He wants a turn.		5
T		Can he go?		3
J		Yeah.	1	
T		How does that work, Jay?		6
J		Gotta [one syllable].	2	
T		Gotta what?		3
J	95a.	*Now her getting off the elevator.	7	
J	95b.	*No, this elevator.	3	

continued

Pragmatics		Speaker	Utterance Number	Dialogue	Morpheme Count		Syntax	Semantics
Child	Adult				Child	Adult		
		T		Uh-huh.		1		
		J	96.	*Bring the other people.	4			
		J	97.	*That doesn't go.	4			
		T		Why not?		2		
		T		What are you doing now?		6		
		J	97a.	The girl wanna go up in. . .(inc.)	—			
		T		Up in. . .?		2		
		J		That her [one syllable]	3			
		J	98.	*Three people.	2			
		J	99.	*That how many.	3			
		J	100.	*The other three people.	4			
		T		What about the little bear?		5		
		J	101.	Gotta sit down.	3			
		T		Why?		1		
		J	102.	'Cause—at home.	3			
		T		At home?		2		
		T		Can he come out to play, too?		7		
		J	103.	No, her mommy say, "No!"	5			
		T		Why?		1		
		J		Because.	1			
		T		The bear says, "I wanna come outside!"		9		
		J	104.	*Then the fire would kill him.	6			
		T		"I'll be real careful."		6		
		T		He says, "How can I get down off this high roof?"		12		
		J	105.	You can jump.	3			
		T		But he might hurt himself.		6		
		T		Can he take the elevator down?		6		
		T		What's he doing?		5		
		J	106.	Trying to put the elevator.	6			
		J	107.	*Her momma home.	3			
		T		And now momma says, "It's time to go to bed."		12		
		T		All the little bears have to go to bed.		10		
		J		Okay.	1			
		T		What's the bear say?		5		
		J	108.	"Me wanna go outside."	4			
		T		Me wanna go outside.		4		

				T		And he calls down to the dog, and what does he say?		14	
			J		108a.	"Doggie, come up and now, okay?"	6		
				T		So, the doggie goes up, and then what happens?		11	
			J		109.	The fire comes up.	5		
				T		How's he gonna get up?		6	
				T		Are they all going to bed?		7	
			J			Yep.	1		
				T		He says, "I don't wanna go to bed yet."		12	
				T		What's mommy say?		4	
			J		110.	"You gotta go to bed right now!"	7		
				T		"No, why?"		2	
				T		"Why do I have to go to bed?"		8	
			J		111.	"Because you naughty!"	3		
				T		"I'm not naughty."		4	
				T		"I put out the fire and saved you."		9	
				T		And he says, "Mommy, when are you going to bed?"		12	
			J		112.	"'Cause, I don't want to."	6		
				T		*When* are you going to bed?		7	
				T		Are they all sleeping?		5	
			J		113.	This guy is.	3		
				T		Is mommy going to let him sleep on top of the roof like that?		15	
			J			No.	1		
				T		What happens if he rolls off the roof when he's sleeping?		15	
			J		114.	He hurt himself.	3		gloss: would hurt
				T		Right, so we better put him to bed.		8	
			J		115.	*Gotta get the girl out.	5		
				T		Gotta get the girl out.		6	
				T		Don't get your hand caught.		6	
			J		116.	*What that fire engine doing up on the roof?	10		
				T		You mean the fireman?		5	
			J			Yeah.	1		

continued

Pragmatics		Speaker	Utterance Number	Dialogue	Morpheme Count		Syntax	Semantics
Child	Adult				Child	Adult		
		T		He's sleeping.		4		
		T		He says, "I'm sleeping; leave me alone."		10		
		J	117.	*They wanna sleep together.	4			
		T		They wanna sleep together.		5		
		T		That's nice.		3		
		T		What if he rolls off?		6		
		J	118.	*I wanna get out now.	5			
		T		You wanna get out now?		6		
		T		How come?		2		
		T		Shhhh! Everybody's sleeping.		4		

[a]*Doesn't* is counted as two morphemes. Following Brown's counting rule #6 (1973, p. 54), the constituent *does* is an irregular verb form that is treated as a single morpheme. The negated form *(n't)* also is treated as a single morpheme, as suggested by Brown (1973, p. 53), ". . . almost every new kind of knowledge increases length (such as) the addition of negative forms. . . ."

[b]*Outta* is not accounted for in Brown's (1973) morpheme counting rules. It is arbitrarily counted here as representing one morpheme.

CHAPTER 4

Exploring Children's Communicative Intents

Robin S. Chapman

Contents

DIVERSITY IN CATEGORIES OF COMMUNICATIVE INTENTS

One branch of work in pragmatics is devoted to the analysis of speakers' communicative intents: the reasons why people talk. The categories developed are diverse, depending on the author's purpose, data, and philosophical point of view. The purpose of this chapter is to summarize some of the taxonomies that seem appropriate for children's language use and to suggest when one might want to use the different systems. One reason for the diversity lies in the different developmental levels of children studied. In this chapter, the taxonomies are grouped according to the ages of the children with whom they have been used, beginning with those used to categorize the first intentional communicative acts of children.

A second reason for the diversity of categories lies in the differing degree to which discourse and social context are considered. At least four levels of analysis are found.

1. *Utterance Level* Many of the taxonomies discussed in this chapter have been developed to classify the speaker's intent at the utterance level, independent of the utterance's function in relation to the prior or subsequent utterance, to the overall discourse structure, or to the social structure of the interaction. If one asks, "What is the speaker doing in uttering this?", without additional information, answers might include *asserting, labeling, promising, warning* or *ordering*. John Searle's (1976) speech act categorization scheme is one example of utterance level categorization. Dore's (1975, 1978) lists include others.
2. *Discourse Level: Utterance Related* One can also categorize the purpose of the same utterance with respect to the previous utterance: does it serve to initiate or continue a topic, answer a question, seek clarification, or acknowledge the other speaker's point? An utterance coded by speech act schemes as *labeling* can also be coded, at this second level, as an *answer* or as an *introduction of a new topic.* With respect to subsequent utterances, an utterance may commit the listener to acknowledgment of the answer or to continuation of the topic.
3. *Discourse Level: Speech Act Related* Not all analyses based on discourse limit themselves to the immediately preceding or following utterance. Considering a still larger framework of analysis—that of *conversational discourse* or *narration,* for example—a third set of discourse functions can be identified for many utterances. They may serve, for example, to open the conversation, to keep the floor, to offer the floor, or to take one's turn. Some speech acts (at the utterance level of analysis) act in the service of other speech acts; for example, requesting attention can be preparatory to requesting action. These latter speech acts are designated *discourse speech acts* (see Garvey, 1975) because they re-

quire a larger unit of analysis for their identification than the utterance alone or the context of immediately preceding and following utterances.

4. *Social Level* Finally, analyses can be placed in the context of the social interaction of the speaker and listener. This may reveal the motivational sources for the communicative intents that have been categorized, as well as an explanation for the forms used in carrying out those intents. In particular, the social obligations to be polite or to be informative often lead to conflicting choices of specific communicative functions, content, and form. One could characterize conversations, then, by the degree to which the participants are primarily concerned to be informative, or polite, or by some other dispositional characteristic associated with cultural conventions.

   Among the schemes available to quantify such judgments are Bales' Social Interaction Scale (1950), Folger and Puck's (1976) rating scheme for dominance using questions and answers, Labov and Fanshel's (1977) detailed discussion of ways to mitigate (soften) or aggravate (sharpen) requests, and James' (1978) scoring scheme for the politeness of children's requests.

A third reason for the diversity found in categories arises from the dimensions used. The basis for coding an utterance at any level may or may not be a pragmatic one in the coding schemes reviewed in this chapter. For example, formal similarity can be the basis of comparing one utterance with another, as is the case for categories such as exact repetition or expansion. If the interclausal semantic relations between utterances are the basis of categorization, categories such as explanation, denial, or justifying may arise (see, for example, Tough's, 1977, coding scheme). Pragmatically based categorization of utterance-related categories includes question-answer sequences, summons and reply, or comment and acknowledgment.

This brief discussion of different levels and dimensions of description is introduced here to alert the reader to the following fact: *there are multiple perspectives from which an utterance's communicative intent may be judged.* Furthermore, the basis of judgment is not always a purely functional one; some researchers distinguish communicative intents primarily by semantic or syntactic characteristics. Almost all the systems reviewed in this chapter attempt to set up mutually exclusive categories, with the implicit notion that each utterance (or, sometimes, propositional unit) will receive a single code. The point made here is that utterances may have multiple, rather than single, communicative intents when viewed from different levels of description or bases of comparison. With that preamble, what follows is a developmentally organized discussion of categories in present use.

CATEGORIES FOR EARLY COMMUNICATIVE INTENTS: SENSORIMOTOR STAGES 4, 5, AND 6 (6 to 24 months)

Early communicative intents have been studied most intensively by Halliday (1975), Dore (1974, 1975), Bates (1976), Bates et al. (1979), and Greenfield and Smith (1976). Bates, in particular, has extended her analysis to nonverbal communicative attempts on the part of the child. Coggins and Carpenter (1978) have adapted Dore's categories for nonverbal children. Ricks (1975) has examined the communicative effect of 8- to 11-month-olds' vocalizations.

The studies typically fail to find examples of intentional communicative vocalization until about 9 to 12 months, or sensorimotor periods Late 4 or Early 5. This correspondence is confirmed when cognitive level is directly assessed (Dihoff and Chapman, 1977).

The category schemes differ primarily in *semanticity,* that is, the degree to which distinctions in semantic content are also captured, and in *discourse level,* the degree to which formal or functional relations to preceding utterances are incorporated in the description. Consider, as you read the following descriptions, which categories are primarily defined by functional intent, which are defined by semantic content, and which are defined by formal or functional relations to preceding or following context.

Differentiated Vocalizations

Ricks (1975) reported that mothers were able to differentiate vocalizations of several different English and non-English babies 8 to 11 months old taped under four different conditions: *request* noises when hungry and shown food; *frustrated* noises when the food was withheld; *greeting* noises upon seeing the mother after a nap or when she returned after an absence; and a *surprised* noise obtained by blowing up a balloon or lighting a sparkler in the baby's presence. There is no evidence that different vocalizations were intended to be communicative by the babies, but their effects were communicative— similarly interpreted—across cultural and linguistic differences. In Austin's (1962) terms, the vocalizations could be called *perlocutionary* for their effect on the listener.

Protoimperatives and Protodeclaratives

Bates (1976) defines two precursors to the first functional uses of speech: the *protodeclarative* and the *protoimperative.* The *protodeclarative* is defined as a preverbal effort to direct the adult's attention to some event or object in the world. Included here are exhibiting the self, showing objects, and pointing or giving sequences in the service of capturing the adult's attention.

The *protoimperative* is defined as the child's use of means to cause the adult to do something. It grows out of more instrumental behaviors in which the child tries to reach the object himself—reaching, opening and closing the hand, intensified cooing sounds. The first protoimperative instances involve these behaviors and, in addition, looking back at the adult. Later, ritualized gesture and vocalization, accompanied by intermittent looking at the adult, would be classified as a protoimperative by Bates, or as a performative by Greenfield and Smith (1976).

Halliday's Functions of Language: Phases I and II

In categorizing the child's early uses of language, Halliday (1975) lists seven functions:

1. The *instrumental,* in which language serves the "I want!" function of seeking satisfaction of material needs
2. The *regulatory,* in which language serves the "Do as I tell you" function, regulating the behavior of others
3. The *interactional,* in which language serves the "me and you" function used in the interaction between the self and others
4. The *personal,* in which language serves the "Here I come!" function used for the direct expression of feelings and attitudes, and for the personal element in interaction
5. The *heuristic,* in which language serves the "Tell me why" function used to investigate reality and to learn about things
6. The *imaginative,* in which language serves the "Let's pretend" function used to create the child's own environment
7. The *informative,* in which language serves the "I've got something to tell you" function used to communicate new information about something

Examples of the four functions that first appeared in his son Nigel's 9- to 10-month speech are given in Table 1. No instances of intentional vocal communication were noted in the preceding 3 months of observation.

Heuristic and *imaginative* uses occurred somewhat later. Examples from Nigel's 16- to 18-month speech are given in Table 2. Halliday points out that by this second phase of Nigel's communicative de-

Table 1. Halliday's (1975) language functions and examples at 9 to 12 months in Nigel (beginning of phase 1)

Function and example	Vocalization	Gloss
Instrumental		
Generalized request for object	/nã/ =	Give me that.
Request for specific object	/bø/ =	Give me that bird.
Rejection of object	light touch of object =	I don't want that.
Regulatory		
General request for action	/ɜ̃/ =	Do that again.
Interactional		
Vocalization upon appearance of person	/ˈdɔ/ =	Nice to see you. Shall we look at this together?
	/na/ =	Anna!
Vocalization in response to other's vocalization	/ɘ:/ =	Yes it's me.
Vocalization in response to gift	/ɛ^{y}a/ =	What's that? There it is.
Vocalization in response to regulation	/a/ =	(loudly) yes?!
Personal		
General interest in participation	/ˈdɔ/ =	Look, that's interesting.
Comment on objects	/ˈdɔ/ =	dog
Expression of pleasure	/ʔn͡ŋ/ =	That tastes nice.
Withdrawal	/g̓^{w}ɤl/---/ =	I'm sleepy.

Source: Halliday, 1975, pp. 148–149.

Table 2. Halliday's (1975) language functions and examples at 16 to 18 months in Nigel

Function and example	Vocalization	Gloss
Instrumental		
Generalized request for object	/m/	= Give me that.
Request for food	*more*	= I want some more.
	cake	= I want some cake.
Request for specific objects or entertainment	*ball*	= I want my ball.
	Dvořak	= I want the Dvořak record on.
	fish	= I want to be lifted up to where the fish picture is.
Regulatory		
General request for action	/ɛ/	= Do that (again).
Specific requests for activity	*book*	= Let's look at a book.
	lunch	= Come for lunch.
Request for permission	*stick-hole*	= Can I put my stick in that hole?
Request for assistance	/ɛ/	= Pick me up (gestures).
Interactional		
Greeting person	/alouha/	= hello
	Anna	
Seeking person	*Anna?*	= Where are you?
Finding person	*Anna*	= There you are.
Initiating routines	*devil*	= You say, "ooh you are a devil."
Expressions of shared regret	/ˀa:/	= Let's be sad; it's broke.
Response to "look"	/m/	= Yes, I see.
Response to *where* question	/de/	= There is it.
Personal		
Comment on appearance of object	*star*	= There's a star.
Comment on disappearance	*no more*	= The star has gone.
Express feelings of:		
interest	/ɸ/	= That's interesting.
pleasure	/ayi:/	= That's nice.
surprise	/o/	= That's funny.
excitement	/ɷ /	= Look at that.
ritual joy	/ɛ/	= That's my ________!
warning	/ɏ :/	= Careful, it's sharp.
complaint	/ɛ:he/	= I'm fed up.
Heuristic		
Request for information	/ʒ$^{\text{ad}^{\text{y}}\text{da}}$/	= What's that called?
Acknowledgment	/m/	= I see.
Imitating	(imitates name)	= It's a ____________.
Imaginative		
Pretend play	(g^{w}ɤl---/	= Let's pretend to go to sleep.
	/ɹa::o/	= Roar; let's pretend to be a lion.
Jingles	*cockadoodledo*	
Rhymes	(supplies final word)	

Source: Halliday, 1975, pp. 156–157.

velopment, he is already combining the basic meaning functions within utterances—for example, observation of an object and demand for it.

From 16 to 35 months, which Halliday identifies as Phase II of language use, two principal functions can be found: the *pragmatic* and the *mathetic*. The older child combines instrumental, regulatory, and interactional functions in what Halliday calls the general *pragmatic* function of speech. This function is defined by the use of the symbolic system to act on reality, that is, the language of request. The interactional, personal, and heuristic functions combine in Phase II in what Halliday calls the general *mathetic* function of speech. In this function, the symbolic system is used as a means of learning about reality or reflecting it. The function is illustrated in the commenting or narrative uses of language.

Finally, informative use of speech, the seventh basic type of use predicted for early utterances, appears during Phase II, at about 22 months in Nigel. For the first time, the child informs the listener about events that are not immediately present and obvious through introduction of topics remote in time or space.

It should be pointed out that ages at which Nigel acquires the different functions may be earlier than the average child's; there is insufficient data on this point. Furthermore, some instances belonging in Halliday's categories are later emerging than the early examples cited. For example, Lezine (1973) reports that novel uses of language in symbolic play to label objects as something different than they are—calling a canteloupe slice an airplane, for example—do not appear until about 24 months, a good many months later than routine conventional use of objects or early pretend play, also categorized as *imaginative* by Halliday.

Greenfield and Smith's Communicative Functions

Greenfield and Smith (1976) distinguish three functional categories in children's earliest communicative vocalizations. The first of these is the *performative* sound accompanying an action. Included here are instances of *Dada* to accompany every action, *Hi* and *Bye-bye* accompanied by waving, and vocalization with pointing. The second and third categories are *indicative* and *volitional performative objects,* emerging in that order. Indicative uses call attention to objects by naming them, accompanied by looking and later by pointing. The volitional category is the demand one; mention of the desired object accompanied by reaching or gesture. The vocative *Mama* accompanied by reaching toward an object would also be an example of a volitional use.

The functional aspects of these categories correspond to routines (or imitation) in the case of pure performatives, to commenting in the case of indicatives, and to requesting an object in the case of volitional uses. The vocalizations accompanying these uses might be general forms (*unh!* accompanying every requesting reach for an object) or the object name. The general form may or may not be interpreted by the mother as a word: compare *unh* plus reaching with *da* plus reaching. The latter is a more likely candidate for morphemic interpretation as *that* by English-speaking mothers.

When differentiated object names appear in this early period, they are initially used to indicate, rather than request, objects. One can argue, then, that a given utterance form in this period is tied to a single function (Ingram, 1971; Halliday, 1975; Greenfield and Smith, 1976; Menn and Haselkorn, 1977). At about 16 to 18 months, this restriction disappears; new vocabulary is used for multiple purposes (Ingram, 1971; Halliday, 1975; Greenfield and Smith, 1976).

Longitudinal Development of the Attention to Object Interaction

Bruner (1978) reports on the longitudinal development of the components of Greenfield and Smith's (1976) indicative and volitional performatives in one child. Interactions in which the child was attending to objects in the presence of the mother constituted the data base.

In the early part of the first year of life, the infant could neither reach nor point toward an object that he wanted or was interested in. He could only cry or fret or look at it. These actions had *perlocutionary* force: the mother behaved as if the child's behavior was purposeful. Most of the first 4 or 5 months of mother-child interaction, however, were spent in looking at one another. Eighty percent of the infant's contact time was spent in looking at the mother's face. Eye contact, smiles, vocalizations, and a variety of exchanges are the characteristic interactions of sensorimotor Stages 1 and 2.

At 4 or 5 months, when the infant was able to coordinate reaching with looking, the face-to-face interaction with the mother dropped to 15% of contact time. Objects preoccupied the child: he reached for them, mouthed, or manipulated them. The mother was not incorporated in his object interactions, although fretting over an object he couldn't reach may have had the effect of getting the mother to obtain it for him. The mother closely monitored what the infant was looking at during this period of object interaction.

By Stage 4, or 8 to 11 months, children are reported to follow consistently the mother's line of regard when it shifts abruptly (Scaife and Bruner, 1975). Thus, joint attention to objects characterizes the mother-child interaction from the beginning of the period in which the child attempts communication (Collis and Schaffer, 1975). The child's reaching at 8 to 10 months has become less effortful. The mother is now incorporated in the child's interaction with the object through gaze shifts; the child looks at the mother and back at the object while reaching.

The indicative reaching gesture then becomes dissociated from the intention to get the object and may only signal an interest in getting the mother to look. The gesture may then be replaced by pointing, accompanied by vocalization and looking back at the mother, to indicate novel or unexpected objects or pictures of familiar objects.

This rather lengthy description makes clear that there are multiple components that must be integrated into early communicative acts, most of them requiring an interactive context for their acquisition.

Dore's Primitive Speech Acts

Dore (1975) defines a set of primitive speech acts identified in the one-word speech of children beginning to talk. These include *labeling, repeating, answering, requesting action, requesting answer, calling, greeting,* and *protesting*. Examples are given in Table 3.

Nonverbal Pragmatic Categories

Coggins and Carpenter (1978) define a set of eight pragmatic categories identifiable in preverbal (or nonverbal) children, based on Dore's (1975) and Bates's (1976) work: *requesting objects, action, or information, greeting, transferring, showing off, acknowledging,* and *answering*. Definitions are listed in Table 4. The requests for action and information listed there are typically later to appear than requests for objects.

Formal versus Functional Categorization

The category of repetition included by Dore (1975) is defined by form rather than by intent. If one wishes to capture the child's communicative purposes, repetition is not a particularly useful category; indeed, it obscures those purposes. But formal similarity of one utterance to a preceding one may nevertheless be important to note for diagnostic purposes: in determining developmental level, in classifying the child as an imitator or not, in accounting for child imitations and the appearance of topic continuation, and possibly in determining the interactional support for early language acquisition. Younger children (Early Stage I linguistically (Brown, 1973); sensorimotor Stage 6) imitate parental speech more frequently than older children (Seitz and Stewart, 1975). These imitations are likely to be of words or semantic rela-

Table 3. Dore's list of primitive speech acts

Speech act	Definition	Example
Labeling	Uses word while attending to object or event. Does not address adult or wait for a response.	C touches a doll's eyes and says *eyes.*
Repeating	Repeats part or all of prior adult utterance. Does not wait for a response.	C overhears Mother's utterance of *doctor* and says *doctor.*
Answering	Answers adult's question. Addresses adult.	Mother points to a picture of a dog and asks *What's that?* C answers *bow-wow.*
Requesting action	Word or vocalization often accompanied by gesture signaling demand. Addresses adult and awaits response.	C, unable to push a peg through hole, utters *uh uh uh* while looking at Mother.
Requesting	Asks question with a word, sometimes accompanying gesture. Addresses adult and awaits response.	C picks up book, looks at Mother, and says *book?* with rising terminal contour. Mother answers *Right, it's a book.*
Calling	Calls adult's name loudly and awaits response.	C shouts *mama* to his mother across the room.
Greeting	Greets adult or object upon its appearance.	C says *hi* when teacher enters room.
Protesting	Resists adult's action with word or cry. Addresses adult.	C, when his mother attempts to put on his shoe, utters an extended scream of varying contours while resisting her.
Practicing	Use of word or prosodic pattern in absence of any specific object or event. Does not address adult. Does not await response.	C utters *Daddy* when he is not present.

Source: Adapted from Tables 1 and 2, Dore, 1975.

tions that the child is in the process of acquiring (Bloom, Hood, and Lightbown, 1974); that is, they appear semantically progressive.

But there is another piece to the puzzle of when these imitations are likely to occur: they are three times as likely to take place if the preceding utterance of the mother is itself a repetition or expansion of the child's utterance (see Table 5 and Folger and Chapman, 1978). This finding suggests that the mother is tuned to the newly developing aspects of the child's repertoire and is more likely to confirm or seek clarification of these newly emerging forms, providing discourse support for repetition or expansion by the child. Thus the formal categories of parent repetition and expansions may be useful in examining the number and semantic contexts of the opportunities for imitation provided to the child; and the degree to which these opportunities give rise to child imitation and expansion may reflect the active process of acquisition.

Table 4. Pragmatic behaviors in nonverbal children

Category	Definition
Requesting	Solicitation of a service from a listener:
Object requests	Gestures or utterances that direct the listener to provide some object for the child
Action requests	Gestures or utterances that direct the listener to act upon some object in order to make it move. The action, rather than the object, is the focus of the child's interest.
Information requests	Gestures or utterances that direct the listener to provide information about an object, action, or location
Greeting	Gestures or utterances subsequent to a person's entrance that express recognition
Transferring	Gestures intended to place an object in another person's possession
Showing off	Gestures or utterances that appear to be used to attract attention
Acknowledging	Gestures or utterances that provide notice that the listener's previous utterances were received
Answering	Gestures or utterances from the child in response to a request for information from the listener

Source: Coggins and Carpenter, 1978.

Functions of Mothers' Speech to Children in Early Stage I

It is also interesting to look at categories of communicative intent in the speech that mothers address to their children. Such a categorization was carried out by Folger and Chapman (1978) for six upper-middle-class mothers talking to their 19- to 25-month-old children (see Table 6). Five of the six children were in Brown's Early Stage I; the sixth in Late Stage I. The speech act scheme was adapted from Dore's (1977) system for older children that is summarized in the next section of the chapter.

What should be noted, in this distribution of speech acts, is that requests for information predominate: about 37% of the total utterances fall in this category. Requests for action comprise 15% of the mothers' utterances on the average; comments (statements and descriptions) 29%; and conversational devices 10%.

Sachs and Devin (1973) have provided a detailed breakdown of the functions of mothers' questions in talking to children (see Table 7). Two-year-olds are more likely than older children to be asked for information about internal states than about the external world. Note that Sachs and Devin were classifying the purposes of utterances that were in question form; thus their list includes a breakdown of requests for action (goods, services, prohibition, attention) as well as a breakdown of requests for information (about external world; internal state; exam questions; requests for permission, approval, confirmation, and clarification). Utterances not in question form that may have served similar purposes were ignored in their breakdown.

Table 5. Mean percentage of parental speech acts imitated by six children ages 1;7 to 2;1 with parent expansions as a separate category (mean age 1;9; Brown's linguistic Stage I)

Parent's utterance	Average percentage imitated	Range
Imitative expansion	32%	10%-46%
Exact repetition	22%	0%-53%
Descriptions	9%	0%-14%
Statements	5%	0%-11%
Requests for information	8%	2%-18%
Requests for action	4%	1%-12%
Conversational devices	2%	0%- 4%

Source: Adapted from Folger and Chapman, 1978, Table 4, page 33.

Table 6. Distribution of 4489 mothers' speech acts to their six children ages 1;7 to 2;1 during free play and lunch settings (mean age 1;9; Brown's linguistic Stage I)

Speech act	Average percentage	Range
Request for information	37.2%	31.4%-44.2%
Request for action	14.9%	10.1%-17.4%
Statements	16.2%	10.0%-23.2%
Descriptions	13.0%	10.3%-15.4%
Conversational devices	9.7%	6.4%-15.1%
Repetitions	2.7%	1.4%- 3.6%
Elicited imitation	0.7%	0.3%- 1.0%
Performative play	1.2%	0.1%- 2.9%
Request for permission	0.2%	0.0%- 0.4%
Other	3.1%	0.3%- 7.8%

Source: Adapted from Folger and Chapman, 1978, Table 2, page 32.

Table 7. Functions of question forms in mothers' speech to children

1. Seeking information about external world
2. Seeking information about internal states
3. Requesting goods
4. Requesting services or prohibiting actions
5. Requesting permission
6. Instruction (eliciting answer to something the speaker already knows)
7. Seeking approval or confirmation
8. Seeking clarification
9. Attention getting

Source: Sachs and Devin, 1973

Summary of Developmental Changes in Early Communicative Intents

Certain functional categories of communicative interaction that are common to all the preceding descriptions of 9- to 12-month-olds can be distinguished: participation in routine games (see also Bruner, 1975a, 1975b; Ninio and Bruner, 1978; Ratner and Bruner, 1978); requesting objects or assistance; rejecting proffered objects or activities; and indicating an object to the mother or commenting on its appearance. These are designated *routines*, *requesting objects or activity*, *rejection*, and *commenting* in Table 8, a reinterpretation of the data from the preceding taxonomic studies.

All four categories appear to have precursors in gestural communication (Bates, 1976; Pea, 1978). The routines usually include an imitative gestural component (Greenfield and Smith, 1976). Requesting is preceded by reaching and looking at the mother, as is commenting. Rejecting is initially accomplished by a pushing-away gesture of the hand with the face averted, and often protesting vocalizations (Pea, 1978).

The major change at approximately 16 to 18 months appears to be the emergence of speech in response to speech: requests for information, usually a request for an object's name; answers to routine *where* and *what's this* and *what does the X say* questions; and acknowledgments of the prior speaker's comment. These are categories of intent that place obligations for talking on the other partner, or that fulfill these obligations. Halliday's heuristic category includes examples of requests for information but the answer category here could cut across many of his functions.

At the end of the sensorimotor period, about 24 months, imaginative uses of language can be de-

Table 8. Summary of developmental sequence of communicative intent in the intentional sensorimotor child

Stage	Intentions
Communicative intents or (sensorimotor Stage 4, 8-10 months)	Routines Gestural precursors to: Requesting objects or activity Rejection Commenting
Utterances expressing communicative intents (sensorimotor Stage 5, or 9-15 months)	Vocal[a] and gestural versions of: Requesting objects or activity Rejection Commenting
Utterances with discourse functions (sensorimotor Stage 6, or 16-22 months)	Discourse functions: Requesting information Answering Acknowledging
Utterances with symbolic function (Early Preoperations, or 24 months on)	Creating reality: Symbolic play Evoking absent objects and events

[a]In most reports, vocalization accompanies the gesture, or has replaced it, by the middle of this period.

tached from objects in symbolic play, when the label *(hat)* creates or transforms the physical object (e.g., plate) (Lezine, 1973; Halliday, 1975). Mention of absent objects or events allows the child, for the first time, to be informative from the listener's point of view. This does not mean, of course, that the child recognizes the conversational obligation to be informative; most of the child's speech is still about content obvious or well-known to the listener. This interpretation of the developmental sequence is summarized in Table 8.

CATEGORIES OF COMMUNICATIVE INTENTS IN THE PREOPERATIONAL PERIOD: 2 TO 7 YEARS

The child's speech from 2 to 7 years becomes complex enough to demand more elaborate differentiation of communicative intent. Utterances begin to reflect not only the basic intents of the sensorimotor period, but also a much wider variety of discourse functions. Form begins to vary with social characteristics of the interactors and settings.

The meanings the child is expressing shift from a here-and-now marking of prevalent semantic roles such as agent, action, and object to speech about interpropositional relations removed in time and space from the conversation. Many of the category schemes of language use developed for preschoolers capture these semantic changes in some detail (e.g., Tough, 1977; Dore, 1978).

In making clinical application of the category schemes developed for this and the next period one needs to sort out when one is looking chiefly at semantic development and when one is seeing changes in communicative intent. Furthermore, one again needs to distinguish categories defined on the basis of formal relations to preceding utterances (e.g., repetition, imitation, expansion) from categories indicating the purposes of those utterances.

The taxonomies summarized in the next section are split into those used chiefly with 2- to 4-year-olds or their parents in the early preoperational period (Sachs and Devin, 1973; Halliday, 1975; Keenan, 1977; Moerk, 1975; Folger and Chapman, 1978; Dore, 1978) and those used with children ages 4 to 7 in late preoperations (Tough, 1977; Garvey, 1977).

Communicative Intents in the Early Preoperational Period

Functions of Language Phase II of Halliday's (1975) scheme for characterizing language use stretched from 16 months to 3 years in Nigel's speech. Examples of utterances found at its beginning were given in Table 2. The seven basic functions of language were usually combined in Nigel's speech, during Phase II, to produce utterances that were primarily *pragmatic* (language for doing) or *mathetic* (language for learning).

Halliday identifies a third, adult phase in Nigel's speech at about 3 years. Now each utterance is multifunctional, reflecting purposes with respect to interaction with the other person *(interpersonal)*; purposes with respect to the forms of the preceding and following utterances *(textual)*; purposes with respect to the expression of meaning *(ideational and experiential)*; and purposes with respect to the social context. Although the seven basic uses of language that Halliday identifies can still be matched to differing social contexts demanding these basic functions, the 3-year-old child is choosing what to say and how to say it for multiple reasons with each utterance: he defines his social relationship with the other, observes and creates discourse obligation, and speaks for purposes consistent with the social setting.

Halliday's view of language function, then, entails 1) a developmental sequence in the emergence of the seven basic functions, 2) reorganizations of the relations between form and function during development, and 3) multiple functions associated with multiword utterances.

Table 9. Categories of child language use in mother-child interaction (20 children ages 1;9 to 5;0)

Child category	Mean percent of total utterances (SD)	Direction of change with increasing MLU
Imitates	5.54% (6.99)	Decrease (r = −0.61)
Asks a question	9.62% (6.88)	Increase and then decrease
Expresses a need	10.81% (5.97)	No change
Answers a question	16.98% (9.02)	Increase and then decrease
Encodes from picture book	8.34% (11.39)	Decrease (r = −0.16)
Describes object or event	6.36% (3.67)	No change
Describes own acts	3.07% (2.17)	No change
Describes a past experience	2.71% (2.41)	Increase (r = 0.57)
Describes his plans	3.43% (2.88)	Increase (r = 0.60)

Adapted from Moerk, 1975

Categories of Teaching Interactions Moerk (1975) identifies nine interactional categories for the child that may provide opportunities to learn language (see Table 9). Together these categories account for an average 65% of 2- to 5-year-old children's utterances in conversations with mothers. Some categories decrease in frequency with increasing language level of the child; others increase, showing consistent change, or are related curvilinearly (see Table 9). Changes in frequency are more closely related to MLU than to age.

Conversational Act Categories Dore (1978) has developed the most elaborate scheme for coding what he calls conversational acts in preschoolers' speech. His categories differentiate utterances on the basis of form, function, semantic content, and conversational contingency. The categories are defined and illustrated in Table 10; see Dore (1978) for examples of application of the coding scheme to transcripts.

An earlier version of the same scheme (Dore, 1977) was used to analyze the utterances of seven children ages 2;10 to 3;7 in peer play. A summary of the distribution of major categories across children's utterances is given in Table 11; a detailed breakdown can be found in Dore (1977). From Table 11 one can see that declarative speech (descriptions plus statements—36%) is far less frequent than the 80%-90% values found in adult-adult conversation. Children address questions to peers much less frequently than mothers question them; requests for action are at similar levels.

Study of the Functions of Repetition in 3-Year-Olds' Speech In Dore's 1975 and 1978 taxonomies there is a response category called "repetition of prior utterance." As noted earlier, this category is based on formal similarity alone, although it frequently appears in lists of communicative functions. The fact is that repetition with prosodic variation may be used for a large variety of functions. Keenan (1977) gives a particularly clear discussion of this fact. She categorized the functions of repetition found in her twins' conversations with each other during their third year. The eleven functions of repetition with respect to prior utterances that she found are listed in Table 12. Thus the category of repetition (or its cousins imitation and expansion) are best replaced with functional categories if one's clinical interest is in the purposes for which the child is speaking. Note that the discourse purposes identified by Dore and Keenan for 3-year-olds are considerably more differentiated than the brief 18-month list constructed earlier. (See Table 8.)

Topic Continuation in Adult-Child Discourse In the 2- to 4-year period a large majority (60–70%) of the child's utterances immediately follow those of the other speaker, at least in adult-child conversation (Bloom, Rocissano, and Hood, 1976). What changes, in these immediately following utterances, is the degree to which the child continues the topic of the preceding utterance (Table 13) and the way that the topic is continued (Table 14). Topic continuations increase from 39% of total utterances at Brown's Stage I, 21 months, to 48% at Stage V, 36 months.

Considering just the topic-related utterances (Table 14), imitations that add nothing new to the topic decrease and expansions of the verb phrase in which something new is contributed increase. A fifth category, in which the topic is expanded and a related topic then introduced, only begins to emerge at linguistic Stage V (3 years), accounting for 5% of the topic continuations.

Scherer and Coggins (in preparation) have looked in detail at the contingencies between four 2-year-old children's topic-continuing discourse functions and the discourse functions in the mother's speech. Children were significantly more likely to assert new information following the mother's request for information than they were to assert new information generally; to clarify an utterance following a request for clarification; to acknowledge an utterance following a request for acknowledgment; and to act in response to a request for action.

Thus the frequency of these four specific requests on the mother's part in speaking to Late Stage I children will affect the degree of coherent discourse and topic continuation seen in conversation with the young child. Remember too that the frequency of expansions on the mother's part is likely to lead to increased imitation, and hence increased topic continuation, on the child's part.

Some of these categories decrease in the mother's speech from 2 to 3 years. Imitations and expansions fall to low (e.g., 3%) rates in mothers' speech to Stage II and later children (Nelson, 1973; Seitz and Stewart, 1975). Requests for action in the mothers' speech decrease significantly from 19% at 23 months (Early Stage I) to 10% at 30 months (Early Stage IV) (Rondal, 1978). At the same time, the proportion of mothers' requests for action accompanied by reasons or queries as to whether the child is willing almost double over the same period from 12% to 22% (Rondal, 1978). Requests for information as a general category appear to remain fairly constant: Baldwin and Baldwin (1973) report 36% of mothers' speech to 3-year-olds to fall into this category. Both Moerk (1975) and Baldwin and Baldwin (1975) report wide variation in this category in mothers' speech.

Table 10. Dore's conversational act categories based on grammatical form, illocutionary function, and conversational contingency

Category	Code	Conversational act	Examples
Requests for information, action, or acknowledgment	RQYN	*Yes/no questions* seeking true-false judgments about propositions	Is he playing with it?
	RQWH	*Wh-questions* seeking factual information (including either-or and fill-in-the-blank questions)	What's that? Where is the bear going?
	RQCL	*Clarification* questions about the content of a prior utterance	What did you say?
	RQAC	*Action requests* seeking that the listener do (or stop doing) something	Why don't you feed him a cow? Get a purple block. Come on. Let's look at this.
	RQPM	*Permission requests*	Can I tie your shoe?
	RQRQ	*Rhetorical questions* seeking acknowledgment from listener to allow speaker to continue	You know what?
Responses to requests	RSYN	*Yes/no answers* supplying true-false judgment	No, he's not playing with it.
	RSWH	*Wh-answers* supplying solicited factual information	Out.
	RSCZ	*Clarifications* supplying the relevant repetition	I said no.
	RSCO	*Compliances* verbally express acceptance, denial, or acknowledgment of a prior action or permission request	Okay.
	RSQL	*Qualifications* supply unexpected information in response to the soliciting question	But I wasn't the one who did it.
	RSRP	*Repetitions* repeat part of prior utterances	
Descriptions of verifiable past and present facts	DSID	*Identifications* labeling objects, events, etc.	That's a barn. John is a boy. There's a big choo-choo.
	DSEV	*Events,* actions, processes, etc. are described	I'm drawing a house.
	DSPR	*Properties,* traits, or conditions are described	That's a bear with a wheel.
	DSLO	*Locations* or direction are expressed	Here's the necklace. I put the dollar in the purse.
	DSTI	*Times* are reported	It happened yesterday.
Statements of facts, rules, attitudes, feelings, and beliefs	STRV	*Rules* express rules, procedures, definitions, facts, etc.	You can't ride the rocket. You have to share.
	STEV	*Evaluations* express attitudes, judgments, etc.	That's right. Good.
	STIR	*Internal Reports* express emotions, sensations, and mental events including intents to perform future acts	I'm tired. I don't think that got the table very clean.
	STAT	*Attributions* report beliefs about another's internal states	He wants to go.
	STEX	*Explanations* express reasons, causes, and predictions	It will fall.
Acknowledgments recognize and evaluate responses and nonrequests	ACAC	*Acceptances* neutrally recognize answers or nonrequests	Yes. Oh.
	ACAP	*Approval/agreements* positively recognize answers or nonrequests	Right. Yes.
	ACDS	*Disapprovals/disagreements* negatively evaluate answers or nonrequests	No. Wrong. I disagree.
	ACRT	*Returns* acknowledge rhetorical questions and some nonrequests, returning the floor to the speaker	Really. Mmm.

Organization devices regulate contact and conversation	ODBM	*Boundary markers* indicate openings, closings, and other significant points in the conversation, e.g., topic switches	Hi. Bye. Okay. By the way.
	ODCA	*Calls* solicit attention	John. Hey!
	ODSS	*Speaker selections* explicitly label speaker of next turn	John. You.
	ODPM	*Politeness markers* indicate ostensible politeness	Thanks. Sorry. Please.
	ODAC	*Accompaniments* maintain verbal contact, typically conveying information redundant with respect to context	Here you are.
Performatives accomplish facts by being said	PFPR	*Protests* register complaints about the listener's behavior	Stop.
	PFJO	*Jokes* display nonbelief toward a proposition for a humorous effect	We throwed the soup in the ceiling.
	PFCL	*Claims* establish rights by being said	That's mine. I'm first.
	PFWA	*Warnings* alert the listener of impending harm	Watch out!
	PFTE	*Teases* annoy, taunt, or playfully provoke a listener	You can't do it.
Miscellaneous	NOAN	*No answer* to questions after 2 seconds of silence	
	UNTP	*Uninterpretable* for unintelligible, incomplete, or anomalous utterances	
	EXCL	*Exclamations* express emotional reactions and other nonpropositional information	

Source: Table 1, Dore, 1978; some examples from Folger and Chapman, 1978.

Decreases are also reported over the 2- to 5-year period in the mothers' modeling of language from picture books, description of the children's actions, and corrective feedback (Moerk, 1975; see Table 9).

Summary of the Early Preoperational Period The most striking changes noted in the child's speech during this period are the increasingly differentiated discourse functions (see Dore, 1978, and Keenan, 1977) and the increasing ability to contribute new information on a topic (Bloom, Rocissano, and Hood, 1976). Topic continuation seems to grow first out of the mother's and the child's early tendencies to repeat and expand each other's utterances and secondly out of early request-response sequences in which the new information that the child is to provide is clearly specified in the mother's request (Scherer and Coggins, in preparation).

Table 11. Distribution of conversational acts in the peer play of seven children ages 2;10 to 3;7

Category		Percent of total
Requests		27.0%
Yes/No and Wh-questions	11.7%	
Action requests	10.0%	
Permission requests	4.7%	
Rhetorical questions	0.6%	
Responses		18.5%
To Yes/No and Wh-questions	10.7%	
Agreement	3.2%	
Compliance	3.1%	
Qualification	1.4%	
Descriptions		22.3%
Statements		13.8%
Conversational devices		5.8%
Performatives		10.8%
Uninterpretable		7.9%
Double coded		5.8%
		100.0%

Source: Dore, 1977

Table 12. Functions of repetition in the conversations of twins from 2;9 to 3;9 years[a]

1. To comment attitudinally
2. To agree with
3. To self-inform
4. To query
5. To answer requests for information appropriately
6. To imitate when specifically requested to do so
7. To make counterclaims
8. To make claims matching those of previous speaker
9. To greet back
10. To reverse the direction (roles) of an order or request for information
11. To request clarification of an utterance

Source: Keenan, 1977
[a]Same form but prosodic aspects may vary.

Table 13. Average distribution of topic continuations in child utterances immediately following adult speech (N = 4)

Mean age	Mean MLU	Utterances immediately following adult speech: Same topic, something new	Same topic, nothing new	Different topic	Total
21 months	1.26	0.21	0.18	0.31	0.70
25 months	2.60	0.33	0.06	0.20	0.59
36 months	3.98	0.46	0.02	0.16	0.64

Source: Computed from Bloom, Rocissano, and Hood, 1976.
400 utterances for each child at each stage are included in the consecutive samples.

Thus, schemes that categorize an utterance's function with respect to discourse as well as its speech act character are particularly useful in the early preoperational period. Developmental changes in topic continuation, also important to note, should be apparent even with severe restrictions in productive syntax or utterance length, as long as comprehension is age-appropriate. For example, the delayed child's one-word utterances may continue the mother's topic through the addition of new information 50% of the time, whereas the expected frequency would be 20% for that syntactic level.

When comprehension as well as production skills are impaired, however, one would expect the development of early preoperational discourse skills to be similarly impaired. In such cases, frequency of communicative attempts, compared to frequency of topic initiations in normal children, and the semantic notions encoded by the child may serve as the best indices to potential communicative and cognitive level. The increasing frustration and misbehavior associated with greatly impaired language comprehension and production skills relative to cognitive level should also be remembered as a diagnostic clue.

Communicative Intents in the Late Preoperational Period

Analysis of Requests for Action Garvey (1975) presents both a speech act and a conversational discourse analysis of requests for action between 36 dyads ages 3½ to 5½ years. She analyzes the conversation for the target illocutionary act of requesting action and carries out a content analysis of the subordinate utterances that demonstrates the children's awareness of preparatory and sincerity conditions governing the speech act. Finally, she asks whether indirect forms that are treated by the listener as requests for action are accomplished through mention of or inquiry about those same preparatory and sincerity conditions. Her study is one of the few to examine the relation of speech acts one to another in conversational sequence; and one of the few to document empirically children's awareness of the conditions governing speech acts.

Garvey defines direct requests for action as imperative in form and containing the explicit propositional content *Future Act (A) of Hearer (H).* The minimal discourse unit that she finds for children's requests meeting these criteria is as follows:

Speaker (S) requests action
Hearer (H) acknowledges request

The domain of discourse across which the request for action is the main or target illocutionary act was optionally extended in the children's conversations in five ways: 1) a preparatory segment, 2) an adjunct to the request, offered either before or after, 3) a subsequent clarification response segment initiated by H, 4) S's reiteration or paraphrase of the request-response sequence, if it failed to bring about H's compliance or acknowledgment, and 5) S's acknowledgment of H's acknowledgment.

In the initial or *preparatory segments* studied by Garvey, S and H might cooperate in a question-answer or comment-response routine in which S

Table 14. Average distribution of topic-related discourse (N = 4)

Mean age	Mean MLU	Categories of topic-related discourse: Yes/No only answers	Expansion	Alternative	Imitation
21 months	1.26	0.11	0.33	0.05	0.47
25 months	2.60	0.29	0.37	0.10	0.16
36 months	3.98	0.26	0.51	0.08	0.05

Adapted from: Bloom, Rocissano, and Hood, 1976.
Categories occurring less than 10% of the time in any sample are omitted. These include social routines, recoding of the adult utterance, and expatiation in which new topics are introduced following continuation of the old topic. Note that topic-continuing Wh-questions did not begin until sometime between 25 and 36 months.

sought to obtain H's attention or to make the propositional content clear to H.

For example:

S: *You see that hammer there?*
H: *Yeah.*
S: Hand it to me.

Either immediately before or after making the request, S might add an *adjunct to the request* that was syntactically independent of the imperative.

For example:

S: Give it to me, *okay?*
S: *That's where the iron belongs.* Put it over there.
S: Roll this tape up for me. *I can't do it.*

These adjuncts accompanied 16% of the direct request sequences studied. When Garvey analyzed their content, the largest number (39%) offered a reason or justification for making the request in one of the following ways.

1. By mentioning the antecedent cause. For example:
   S: Stop it. *You hurt my head.*
2. By stating a relevant normative consideration. For example:
   S: Get that off you. *You girls aren't men like that.*
3. By stating the future goal that the request served. For example:
   S: *We have to get all bungled up.* Put it on your head.
4. By stating a need or desire for the action. For example:
   S: Gimme. Gimme that. *I need that.*
5. By stating a desire for an outcome of the action. For example:
   S: Hey, come here. *I want to show you something.*

The second most frequent purpose of these adjuncts (26% of the total) was to query the willingness of H to do A. For example:

S: Here, do that. Do the rest of that, *okay?*

In analyzing children's acknowledgments of a speaker's requests, Garvey found that verbal acknowledgment *(all right, okay)* almost always accompanied compliant behavior, which occurred about 50% of the time. In addition, H might report the accomplishment of the act or elaborate on the propositional content of the request. For example:

S: Just start the motor, okay?
H: *Okay.* (Makes motor noises). *It's started.*
S: Call up a good guy.
H: *I will, I'll call a doctor.* (Lifting receiver).

When H acknowledged the request but verbally postponed fulfilling it, *S* usually took this for compliance and waited. For example:

S: Come on, get on.
H: As soon as I finish putting out this roaring fire. (Plays fireman).
S: (Waits)
H: (Comes to car).

H might also query S's reason for the request rather than comply. For example:

S: Get in here.
H: *How come?*

Finally, in acknowledging S's request H might refuse outright. Typically, the children making a request did not find H's simple refusal *(No!)*, the statement that H was not obliged to *(I don't have to)*, not willing to *(I don't want to)*, or not the appropriate person to *(No, you!)* a sufficient reason for not complying and persisted in repeating or paraphrasing the original demand. Nor did S abandon his request when H asserted his own prior rights or conflicting claims. Those responses of H that were more successful in dissuading S were as follows:

1. Indicating his inability to do A. For example:
   S: Here, do that. Do the rest of that, okay?
   H: *I can't.*
2. Indicating that he does not need or want the outcome of A. For example:
   S: Wait for the snake to come.
   H: *I don't need the snake.*

These findings suggest that the children see the following as conditions for requests for action:

1. S has a good reason for making the request.
2. H is able to do A.
3. H will comply or have a good reason not to.

There is sometimes a dispute between the parties over what constitutes a good reason for asking on the one hand, or refusing, on the other.

Preparatory condition (2), that H be able to do A, matches one of the preparatory conditions that Searle (1969) ascribes to adult requests for action. The other characteristics of the adult conditions are not so clearly revealed in the children's interactions. The sincerity condition—that S wants H to do A—is not explicitly mentioned in the adjuncts and acknowledgments accompanying requests for action. What is mentioned frequently in justifying requests is that S wants A, or its outcome. The preparatory condition that S assumes that H is willing to do A is often cited by unwilling Hs, but rejected as a sufficiently good reason by Ss. The third precondition of successful adult requesting—namely that it not be obvious to both S and H beforehand that H intended to do A—was not mentioned, but neither is it clear that it was ever violated.

It would appear that individual children's understanding of the preconditions governing felicitous requests for action can best be assessed from the conversation when the request (or the response) goes wrong in some way, as when the requesting partner violates one of the putative preparatory or sincerity conditions, or when the listener challenges the speaker on one of these grounds.

Knowledge of the more general conditions governing cooperative conversation can be similarly assessed in probing for the optional segments of the request sequence that establish attention to the speaker, comprehension of the referents, and clarification of the message.

Finally, one may study the child's growing understanding of the discourse obligations carried by a request for action by observing whether he consistently supplies an acknowledgment of the request, as H, or demands one, as S.

Functions of Language Tough (1977) identifies four major functions of language use—directive, interpretative, projective, and relational—in the speech of 3-year-olds, 5½-year-olds, and 7½-year-olds. The specific uses are summarized, with examples from the 3-year-olds, in Table 15.

There one can see that Tough has been primarily concerned with the roles that language plays in problem-solving and thinking. Many of the strategies summarized in Table 15 reflect cognitive changes in children's ability to control their own behavior, to reason, to relate events to one another, and to engage in complex imaginative play.

The examples include many instances of complex language, although one could often infer the same purposes by attending to semantic relations between one-word utterances. The 4-year-old hearing-impaired child with an MLU of 1.2 who says "Paint all done. Home. TV." is using limited language for the advanced cognitive purposes outlined by Tough. Thus her system is valuable for the cognitively advanced semantic content it captures, although it would reveal almost nothing of the child's growing discourse skills.

Table 16 summarizes the language uses of very high IQ English 3-year-olds from advantaged and disadvantaged backgrounds in conversations with a peer and an adult observer. The two groups differed in how they used language, with the advantaged group more likely to use speech in imaginative contexts or to comment on future or past events. The disadvantaged children, in contrast, were more likely to use language to express needs, monitor

Table 15. Tough's framework for the classification of uses of language

Function	Uses	Strategies	Examples from 3-year-olds	
Directive	1. Self-directing	i. Monitoring actions	Jimmie:	(accompanying his actions) This car goes down here. . . the little car. Pushing it down here. . . the little car. All down here. . . pushing it down here. . . pushing it down here . . . la. . . la. . . la.
		ii. Focusing control	Jane:	(trying to turn on the small, stiff taps of the toy bath) Having a bath, and I'm . . . turning. . . it, turning. . . it. It won't turn. (Actions accompany each word).
		iii. Forward planning	Jim:	(planning what he will do next) I am going to cut the clay to make two bits. . . the same. . . then I'll flatten them out. . . well one goes at each end.
	2. Other-directing	i. Demonstrating	Tim:	(demonstrating the actions he requests) Put your car in there like that. That's right. . . now *you* put a brick at the door like this.
		ii. Instructing	James:	Put your brick right on top. Be careful. . . don't push it. . . go and get a flag now. . . fasten it on top with a slide.
		iii. Forward planning	James:	You'll have to get another piece. . . a white one and little and then you'll have to put a pin in the box over there. . . to fasten it on with.
		iv. Anticipating collaborative action (self and other)	Peter:	(to Tom, who is building a wall as Peter drives his car around) There's going to be a crash. . . build yours up high now then we can make them crash together.

Interpretative	1. Reporting on present and past experiences	i. Labeling	Mark:	That's a cowboy and that's an Indian. There's a see-saw...
		ii. Elaborating detail	James:	(Talking about visit to the seaside) We went in the sea...and it was cold...and it splashed. There was a lot of little things...I saw them...little fishes swimming.
		iii. Association with earlier experience and comparison	John:	I've got one of those...but it's not like that one...my one's not got an Indian in it like that.
		iv. Recognizing incongruity	Tom:	The garage is too small for the car to go in.
		v. Awareness of sequence	Jane:	And we went on a holiday...and I was poorly with measles. Then Bobby got the measles...but we're all better now.
	2. Reasoning	i. Recognizing dependent and causal relationships	Jane:	And the ice cream was all soft 'cos we forgot to put it in the fridge.
		ii. Recognizing a principle or determining conditions	Andrew:	People don't like you if you take their things...I don't do that.
Projective	1. Predicting	i. Forecasting events	Mary:	My dad's going to make me a see-saw...when it's summer he's going to.
		ii. Anticipating consequences	Meg:	My mom'll be cross 'cos I've got my sleeves wet.
		iii. Surveying possible alternatives	James:	Well we could go on a bus or a train to my auntie's. I don't know which.
		iv. Forecasting related possibilities	Peter:	(looking at a paperweight snowstorm) If it's got a crack in it the water might come out.
		v. Recognition of problems and predicting solutions	Adrian:	It won't fasten on now it's broked... it won't pull it either. I think some string would do...some string can mend it.
	2. Empathetic	i. Projecting into experiences of others		
		ii. Projecting into other people's feelings	Jane:	She doesn't like Terry teasing... that's horrible...and she's crying 'cos she didn't like it.
		iii. Anticipating the reactions of others		
	3. Imagining	i. Renaming	John:	(Putting two small boxes on the floor): That's for a house where the man lives...and that's ones for the car... a garage.
		ii. Commentary on imagined context	Jill:	(Using an imaginary phone) My baby's poorly...doctor...will you come quickly...will you give her a prick thing to make her better.
		iii. Building scene through language		
		iv. Language of role (includes use of directive and interpretative functions in the imagined context)	Dan:	(Pretending to take the washing around to imaginary ladies). Here you are Mrs....here's your washing...money please...thank you.
Relational	1. Self-maintaining	i. Expression of need		Watch me, see what I'm doing.
		ii. Protection of self-interest		Go away—you're hurting me.
		iii. Justifications		I want a red crayon so I can draw my picture better.
		iv. Criticisms		I don't like your picture.
		v. Threats		Give me a sweet or I'll hit you.
	2. Interactional	i. Self-emphasizing strategy		Give me it that car it's mine.
		ii. Other-recognizing strategy		Would you give me my car back now please 'cos I'm going home.

Source: Adapted from Tough, 1977, pages 68-69; examples from pages 45-67.

their own actions, and identify present objects and events. The uses of 5½- and 7½-year-olds are unfortunately not easy to summarize because their occurrences in standard eliciting situations were not consistently reported by Tough (1977).

The changes with age appeared to consist of an increase in the categories least frequent in the disadvantaged 3-year-olds and somewhat more frequent in the advantaged 3-year-olds. This suggests that the difference in the high and low SES groups may have been in general developmental level despite the initial equating of IQ; and indeed, upon retest at 5½ and 7½ years of age, this proves to be the case (IQs decrease more for the low socioeconomic group than the high).

If the differences can be attributed to the different socioeconomic backgrounds in language use and corresponding syntactic complexity, rather than general developmental level, then Tough makes the interesting suggestion that the differences can be traced to the language uses modeled by the preschoolers' parents. That is, children in the later preoperational period learn to talk about the topics that their parents introduce, and in the way that their parents discuss them. Concomitant differences in MLU and structural complexity, then, may simply reflect the differing uses to which children are putting their language, rather than different levels of structural acquisition. Only additional research in this area can show to what extent the differences that Tough observed arise from either patterns of language use differentially modelled by parents or from differing levels of cognitive and language skill.

Requests for Clarification Garvey (1977) presents a very useful breakdown of the different kinds of contingent query, or requests for clarification, that occur in conversational interaction. One may nonspecifically request repetition of the prior speaker's utterance, specifically request some portion of the utterance, or specifically request confirmation or additional specification. Examples of these types of contingent query are given in Table 17; some other categories discussed by Garvey but not studied in children are omitted here. Note the subtle differences in type of query depending on falling versus rising intonation in Wh-questions; the usual Wh-question is asked with a falling intonation.

For the most part, 3- to 5-year-olds use and answer these four kinds of contingent queries appropriately (see Table 17). Three-year-olds' responses to requests for repetition are the exception. Specific re-

Table 16. Uses of language by high IQ 3-year-olds from high and low socioeconomic backgrounds (Mean Stanford Binet IQ = 129 and 126, respectively; N = 24 for each group)

Use	Socioeconomic Level	
	High	Low
Self-monitoring (i.e. needs status defined)	6%	14%
Directive		
1. Monitoring own actions	8%	29%
2. Extending action and collaborating	3%	1%
Interpretative		
1. Present		
a. Identifying	12%	27%
b. Extension through reference to detail	11%	6%
c. Logical reasoning	4%	1%
2. Past		
a. Identifying	2%	0%
b. Extension through reference to detail	2%	0%
c. Toward logical reasoning	1%	0%
Projective total	52%	21%
1. Predictive	7%	3%
2. Empathetic	0%	0%
3. Imaginative		
a. Directive	14%	9%
b. Extending actions	20%	3%
c. Identifying, representation	2%	2%
d. Extension of imagined context	4%	1%
e. Toward logical reasoning	2%	0%
f. Role taking	2%	3%

Computed from Tough, 1977, page 190, Table 5.
Sample taken during 1-hour play periods with peer and adult observer.

Table 17. Types of unsolicited contingent query among peers in two 15-minute samples (Examples are in response to "Joe Glick knows a friend of yours")

Category	Code	Example	Mean for Dyad			Appropriate Response (percent)		
			3 years (N = 12)	4 years (N = 12)	5 years (N = 24)	3 years (N = 12)	4 years (N = 12)	5 years (N = 24)
Nonspecific request for repetition	NRR	Q. *What?* or *Huh?* A. (Repeat Utterance)	3.33	5.00	4.00	60	90	95
Specific request for repetition	SRR	Q. *A what?* A. A friend of yours	0.33	0.17	0.17	50	100	75
	or	Q. *Who?*↑ A. Joe Glick						
Specific request for confirmation	SRC	Q. *He does?* A. Yes	2.50	3.25	1.25	85	79	73
Specific request for specification	SRS	Q. *Who?*↓ A. That Greek fellow	1.17	1.17	1.54	79	86	86

Source: Garvey, 1977

quests for repetition are rare throughout the samples.

Garvey's categories allow one to differentiate requests for clarification in specific detail. They may prove particularly useful in analyzing the abilities of children to seek information when the message is unclear or to give the clarifying information requested by the listeners. The frequency of these queries would be expected to vary with the intelligibility and referential clarity of the conversationalists, as well as with the discourse skill of the listener. Very little is known about the course of conversation with unintelligible children, but categories such as these may help to study it.

ADULT USES OF SPEECH

Taxonomy of Speech Acts

In extending Austin's (1962) work on how adults do things with words, Searle (1976) proposes five major categories of speech acts. There are *representations* (statements that can be characterized as true or false), *directives* (the speaker attempts to get the hearer to do something), *commissives* (commit the speaker to some future action), *expressives* (express a psychological state), and *declarations* (saying makes it so). These major groupings differ in whether their essential point is to get the world to match the speaker's words *(directives, commissives, declarations)*, to get the words to match the world *(representations, declarations)*, or neither *(expressives)*.

Speech act categories or groupings also differ in their preparatory and sincerity conditions: those beliefs, wants, or intentions on the part of the speaker and hearer that are necessary for the act to be felicitous, or successful. A sincere *representation*, for example, can occur only if the speaker believes that what he or she asserts about the world is true. Preparatory conditions might include the ability to carry out the action and a context in which it is not obvious to both that the hearer will carry out the action in the normal course of events. A sincere *commissive*, for example, only occurs if the speaker actually intends, at the time of speaking, to carry out the future action to which he commits himself. Preparatory conditions may include beliefs about whether the hearer wants—or doesn't want— the action carried out.

Within each of these five major groupings of speech acts are many instances, differing somewhat in their required propositional content, preparatory conditions, sincerity conditions, and essential point. Some examples are listed in Table 18; the analyses of individual speech acts come from Searle (1969).

Learning to Be Clear and to Be Polite

Finally, two very general sets of conditions on speech acts in conversation have been described: the obligation to be clear and informative (Grice, 1975) on the one hand, and to be polite (Lakoff, 1973) on the other. Table 19 summarizes these general conventions that appear to govern speech acts among middle class Standard American English speakers. Different cultures value informativeness and politeness differently; it may be so important to make the other person feel good (Rule 3 of politeness) that the truth of one's assertion (the sincerity condition) is irrelevant. Or information may be a resource that one is unwilling to share; the question-answering of many politicians suggests that this rule of the game is altered by public life.

The observance, or the deliberate violation, of these rules (or a modified, culturally appropriate set) constitutes another set of reasons for which skilled conversationalists talk—to communicate their perceptions of the social relationships and the contexts of the exchange.

The specific and general conditions on speech acts summarized in this section are useful to keep in mind when something seems to have gone wrong in the conversation. Ask if the event triggering a "Tilt" message for the listener was the failure to observe one of these preconditions.

PROBLEMS IN USING THE TAXONOMIES

Confusions of Level

In an earlier section, communicative intents were identified at any of four levels of analysis: utterance, interactive, discourse, and social levels. In practice, many of the existing taxonomies include categories from different levels of analysis, and the opportunity for multiple coding of an utterance from each level's perspective is not always made apparent. One may resolve these ambiguities in two ways—either by adopting a classification scheme as given, so that one's data are comparable, or by systematically altering the available taxonomies to allow coding at the single or multiple levels of clinical interest.

Inferring Intent

A second problem encountered in developing or using taxonomies of communicative functions is that intentions are not observable. Objective criteria for

Table 18. Examples of conditions governing speech acts

Condition	Category (Speech Act)				
	Assertive Statement	Directive (Request)	Commissive (Promise)	Expressive (Congratulate)	Declaration (Resign)
Propositional content	Any verifiable proposition *(p)*	Future act *(A)* of *H*	Future act *(A)* of *S*	Some event *(E)* related to *H*	Termination of employment of *S*
Preparatory conditions	1. Speaker *(S)* has evidence or reasons for the truth of *p* 2. It is not obvious to both *S* and hearer *(H)* that *H* knows *p*.	1. *H* is able to do *A*. 2. *S* believes that *H* is able to do *A*. 3. It is not obvious to both *S* and *H* that *H* will do *A* in the normal course of events of his own accord.	1. *H* would prefer *S*'s doing *A* to his not doing *A*. 2. *S* believes that *H* would prefer his doing *A* to his not doing *A*. 3. It is not obvious to both *S* and *H* that *S* will do *A* in the normal course of events.	1. *E* is in *H*'s interest. 2. *S* believes that *E* is in *H*'s interest.	1. *S* is employed 2. *S* has the authority to terminate his employment same setting that day.
Sincerity rule	*S* believes *p*.	*S* wants *H* to do *A*.	*S* intends to do *A*	*S* is pleased at *E*.	None
Essential rule	Counts as an undertaking to the effect that *p* represents an actual state of affairs.	Counts as an attempt to get *H* to do *A*.	Counts as an undertaking of an obligation to perform *A*.	Counts as an expression of pleasure at *E*.	Counts as an act of terminating the employment of *S*

Source: Searle, 1969, 1976

Table 19. Cooperative principle of conversation. Make your contribution as required in accord with the accepted purposes and direction of the talk exchange.

Be clear[a]	Be polite[b]
Quantity: Informativeness	
1. Make your contribution as informative as required	1. Don't impose on listener
2. Be no more informative than required	2. Give options
Quality: Sincerity condition	3. Make the listener feel good: be friendly
1. Do not say what you believe to be false	
2. Do not say that for which you lack adequate evidence	
Relation: Topic management	
1. Be relevant	
Manner: How to be clear	
1. Avoid obscurity of expression	
2. Avoid ambiguity	
3. Be brief	
4. Be orderly	

[a]Source: Grice, 1975
[b]Source: Lakoff, 1973

these categories are not always easy to develop. Although members of the same cultural and linguistic community may agree in their interpretations, this fact does not guarantee that the speaker intended the same interpretation. Analyses made by clinicians or experimenters who are not members of the speech community of the conversationalists may be particularly suspect, and should be checked with members of that community.

It is possible, of course, to support the inference of intent through collateral evidence: to observe, for example, that the speaker accepts listener interpretations matching one's own categorizations and protests the listener interpretations that do not match. The effect of the speaker's utterances on the listener is another useful kind of collateral evidence, although the effect is not always, of course, what was intended. In the case of infants, in fact, intentional communication may develop out of experiencing the consistent perlocutionary effects of one's *non*communicative activity.

Developmental Changes in the Range of Communicative Intents That Can Be Inferred

A third problem in analyzing communicative intents arises because the basis for inference changes as the syntactic and semantic complexity of a child's utterances increase. Some categories—particularly those finely differentiated with respect to semantic content, (e.g., Dore's description of location) or those dependent upon the use of specific vocabulary (e.g., promising)—may not be identifiable in children at the one- or two-word level. Use of such categories when there is a known restriction or delay in the child's semantic or syntactic production is inappropriate, because it will simply reflect the problems already identified in the child's syntax or semantics. For such children it is important that the functional categories chosen for analysis can be inferred from one word—or even nonverbal—conversational participation. The limitation of this approach, of course, is that many of the developmentally later speech act categories at the utterance level are then excluded from analysis. However, by categorizing communicative intent at the other levels of analysis—interactive, discourse, and social—one may obtain a clearer picture of the child's communicative competence independent of his production skills.

Distinctions Made on Semantic or Syntactic Bases Only

A point to consider in selecting a set of categories for clinical use is that some systems differentiate categories principally on the basis of message content (e.g., Dore's, 1978, description of possession versus description of location) or on the basis of message form (e.g., Dore's 1975 Repeating), rather than message function. The semantic or syntactic characteristics of the utterance may or may not be important to capture clinically; but the clinician should be aware that these aspects, rather than the functional ones, may be reflected by a category system.

The clinical consequences of using a "pragmatic" coding scheme that depends chiefly on semantic (e.g., Tough's 1977 system) or on semantic and syntactic criteria (much of Dore's 1978 system) are: 1) that one will identify as "pragmatically" different children with semantic or syntactic delays; and 2) that one will miss some children with pragmatic differences whose semantics and syntax are normal.

Multiple Functions of an Utterance at the Same Level

Even when the questions of level and content to be coded have been decided, problems in multiple coding may arise in categorizing utterances. This is so because the basic unit of analysis at the different levels is really something corresponding more closely to an underlying *proposition* than to an utterance. For example, the utterance "Hey Jim, find the red ball, okay?" contains (at the utterance interactional level) at least a request for attention, a request for action, and a request for information about the other's willingness to comply.

If one were analyzing this utterance from the perspective of discourse, one would identify the request for action as the main purpose of the speaker and analyze the request for attention and request for information about willingness to comply as preparatory to the request for action. Further analysis at this level would require more of the conversational context; the point here is that multiple categories would have been assigned to the same utterance.

At the level of the social interaction matrix, one would note the informality of speech *(Hey)* suggesting solidarity or equal status; the use of first name in address, suggesting equal or higher status of the speaker; the use of imperative form for requesting action (again suggesting equal or higher status of the speaker); and a polite softening of the request *(Okay?)* suggesting that the speaker is not in a position to order the other around. Again, the point is that there are multiple linguistic choices in a single utterance that may have conventional social significance.

At the utterance level, the example presupposes that a red ball exists, that the listener's name and the particular ball being talked about are already known to the listener, and that he is able to carry out the requested activity and directs him to carry out the same activities listed at the interactional level (attend, act, and reply). Halliday (1975) recognized this multiplicity of functions in a multiword utterance by defining more general functions as the pragmatic and mathetic that incorporated a number of one-word functions; but even these categories are not sufficient to account for more complex utterances, as Halliday himself points out.

Reliability of Categorization Schemes for Communicative Intent

There are almost no data available on the reliability of the coding schemes previously reviewed. Clinical experience in use of many of the systems, however, has suggested that problems are likely to arise in application. The first moral here is plain: clinicians should check their own reliability in using whatever category scheme for communicative intent they have selected. If reliability is low, several questions may be useful to ask in troubleshooting the problem.

Sufficient Information about Context? A first question is whether sufficient information is available about context to make the judgments required. Notes from direct observation or videotape may be necessary to supplement transcripts of conversation. This is particularly true when speech is limited.

Overlapping Categories? A second problem leading to unreliability may be inherent in the category scheme itself. The codes may not be mutually exclusive, or fairly detailed decision rules may be required to make them mutually exclusive when some are subsets of others.

Shifting Levels? If the level of description switches from one category to another (e.g., from utterance level to discourse level and back), clinicians may find themselves attempting to continue to code at a given level when the scheme makes only a few categories available at that level.

Categories Too Detailed for the Available Information? When categories that make fine differentiations on the basis of semantic content are used with younger children, or with children whose productive language is delayed, clinicians may find themselves unable to assign utterances to categories. This too will lead to poor reliability.

Too Many Categories or Too Little Practice? The number of different categories that can be kept in mind will vary with the task (on-line, or opportunity for review) and amount of practice in using the categories. One should make sure that one has sufficient practice in the coding task before evaluating reliability. If reliability continues to be a problem, the solution may lie in reducing the number of coding categories. On-line decisions, in particular, may be easier. A problem inherent in this solution is that categories of quite different intent may be collapsed together. One needs to be sure that the simplified set can be meaningfully interpreted.

Difficulty in Inferring Intent? When intent is difficult to infer even with the aid of context, the uncertainty will directly affect reliability of coding. Here additional training or even a different category scheme may be of little help. The remedy must be sought in the way the communication sample is collected. Has one sampled interactions in which clear communication needs arise for the child? Do the available play materials permit a wide variety of topics and aid the viewer in understanding conversation on those topics? Does the sample include interaction with people familiar with the child, who may be more successful in interpreting his or her intent? Does the interactor check his or her own interpretations with the child, so that evidence from the child's subsequent behavior can be taken into account? Such questions lead one to sample multiple interactions for multiple purposes with multiple topics.

WHEN TO USE WHICH TAXONOMY?

There are several important points to remember in choosing any one of these schemes, or others, for assessment purposes:

1. There are developmental changes in the communicative intents expressed by a child; categories appropriate to developmental levels should be chosen. Cognitive growth may be the closest correlate of these changes in mentally retarded children.
2. There are developmental changes in the form in which communicative intents are conveyed. Development of gross motor and speech motor control mechanisms will affect the emergence of these forms. Thus, categories based on form may mislead one as to the developmental level of pragmatic functioning in children with speech motor control problems or productive syntactic delays.
3. A number of more complex functional characteristics of speech require multiword utterances for their identification. The functions summarized for the sensorimotor child do not, but are developmentally limited. The clinician may have to construct his or her own list when speech production is limited.
4. There may be developmental change or individual differences in the purposes for which mothers talk that give rise to the apparent developmental change or individual differences in the way children talk. The contribution of the other participant to the picture of pragmatic functioning in the child must be evaluated.

The question that one particularly wants to ask should be the first reason for using one of the preceding taxonomies, or inventing one. That question will depend in part on the developmental level of the child and on the expressive means at his command. In the language disordered or delayed child, these two levels may differ.

A number of the systems summarized were developed with children at preverbal or one-word stages: Halliday (1975), Bates (1976), Dore (1975), Greenfield and Smith (1976), Coggins and Carpenter (1978). For a child functioning at sensorimotor Stages 4, 5, or 6 these systems are especially useful. For children in a one-word stage whose cognitive levels of functioning are suspected to be preoperational or more, one needs to supplement these sensorimotor-based taxonomies with lists constructed for children of the appropriate developmental level, selecting just those categories that can be identified on the basis of context and gesture, or *one*-word speech.

None of these taxonomies is exhaustive of the possible functions at all four levels of analysis although some of the one-word ones are intended to be. In older children the use of only one level of analysis may be seriously misleading, failing to reflect the child's growth in constructing multifunctional utterances in the way described by Halliday (1975).

ALTERNATIVE APPROACHES TO EXPLORING COMMUNICATIVE INTENT: WITH ALL THESE PROBLEMS, WHAT IS THE CLINICIAN TO DO?

The preceding coding schemes could, of course, simply be used to quantify free-speech samples in a variety of contexts: that is, to note what the child usually does. Up to this point such uses have been the main focus of attention. Detailed problems in validity and reliability that may arise have already been pointed out. Just as serious a limitation is the fact that only a few of the existing schemes for children beyond 2 years capture developmental change in their present forms. Thus, even a valid and reliable coding scheme may yield relatively little information about the child's developing communication skills, beyond the conclusion that he has a variety of them.

What is the clinician to do? Here, as in other areas of language assessment, the answer seems to lie in taking on an active and probing role in drawing inferences about the child's communication system. Three pieces of advice, in particular, can be offered: 1) take the contexts of communication into account, 2) use discourse rather than utterance levels of analysis for the older child, and 3) evaluate the child's observances and understanding of the *rules* governing speech acts, rather than simply counting instances of speech acts.

Analyze Communicative Intents Relative to Obligatory Contexts

One useful principle is to consider how often an event happens relative to how often it should or could have happened; that is, to define contexts that require (or permit) a given communicative category to occur. These relative frequencies of occurrence are more informative than simple frequency counts. For example, the proportion of requests for action in a speech sample may vary more with the selected activity than with developmental level. But if one considers all the incidents in which the child is attempting to alter another's behavior (including those involving nonverbal confrontation), one could quantify the extent to which a child's communicative intents are verbally realized. Developmental change is to be expected in such a variable, and its relevance to intervention programming becomes plain.

Further, one could code the effectiveness of the child's nonverbal and verbal requests for action, and seek additional ways to help him communicate effectively. Such an approach would require taking nonverbal gestural (see e.g., Lewis, 1978) and social skills, as well as verbal ones, into account.

Finding obligatory contexts—for example, deciding whether or not a child wants to request an object or action at each moment in time—may prove time-consuming and difficult. An alternative approach is to arrange standard eliciting contexts for the basic communicative intents of interest: situations likely to lead to requests for objects or actions, comments, or requests for information. Ricks (1975) used this approach in his collection of infant vocalizations. Snyder (1975) has used it successfully to evaluate early communicative intents in normal and retarded children. Arranging an eliciting context may be especially useful for the very young child who attempts communication infrequently.

Use Discourse Levels of Analysis for Children Beyond 18 Months

A problem with analyses carried out only at the utterance level, even if corrected for obligatory or permitting contexts, is that they reflect nothing of the child's growing skill in discourse. All the interactive information about the conversation is lost. This problem is serious for analyses of children functioning at 18 months and older because the chief developmental change in pragmatic skills of these preschoolers appears to lie in the acquisition of conversational skill. Thus categories reflecting discourse levels of analysis, either related to immediately adjacent utterances or to larger discourse stretches, should be used with preschool level children. For the child beyond 3½ years, the larger discourse context may be the only level at which developmental change is clearly proceeding.

When one uses discourse level categories and, in addition, takes obligatory context into account, one constructs clinically useful and developmentally diagnostic pictures of the child. The clinician may want to know answers to questions such as the following: What proportion of mother's questions are answered by the child? What proportion of her initiated topics are continued by the child? How is topic continuation managed—by repetition, by acknowledgment, or by addition of information? What proportion of the time does the child go on to produce a related topic?

The child's effectiveness as a communicator with peers or adults can also be evaluated. For example, what proportion of the child's questions is answered by the other participant? What proportion of his topics continued? What proportion of the child's requests for action complied with?

These questions permit the clinician to quantify the child's conversational skills as they change over time, and to examine the relations between communicative intent, the way in which communicative intent is carried out, and the speaker's communicative effectiveness. The work of Bloom and her colleagues on topic (Bloom, Rocissano, and Hood, 1976) and the work of Garvey (1975) on requests for action are two of the few examples of this important approach to the child's developing discourse skills.

Evaluate the Child's Rules Governing Speech Acts

A simple counting of speech acts in a speech sample may reveal relatively little about the preschooler's pragmatic skills, although it may be a useful means of comparing the effects of activities and topics on the speech samples obtained. There may be some speech acts, of course, that emerge relatively late: promising, for example. But a counting of instances tells the clinician or researcher nothing about the child's growing mastery of the rules or conventions governing speech acts.

For example, does the child recognize the sincerity condition governing assertions? This can be inferred if the child recognizes the humor of a mislabeling game, or if the child plays it himself as a game. Such games often arise spontaneously around 2 years of age between parent and child: the child giggling and calling mother *Daddy* or father *Mommy* as the parent protests (Davison, 1974). Similarly, playful use of the sincerity conditions governing other speech acts would be naturally-occurring markers of the child's appreciation of the conventions. When a rule is appreciated, its violation can be the subject of humor: here is one basis for the 4-year-old's gleeful use of words he recognizes to be impolite in some contexts.

There has been little study of the child's versions of rules governing speech acts (Garvey, 1975, is an exception), or how the child's rules change; but these are topics whose exploration will repay researchers, clinicians, and children alike. It is through shared knowledge of the implicit conventions governing speech acts and conversational sequence that adults understand each other; and it is the child's growing awareness of the conventions that will signal, and determine, his or her conversational skills.

SECTION II

ELICITING PRODUCTIVE LANGUAGE

This section has two chapters containing procedures directed toward prompting the child to produce utterances of specified form and content. Chapter 5 lists procedures by which linguistic, conversational, and physical context are manipulated to increase the probability that the child will produce the target utterances. The procedures listed in Chapter 5 should be considered as examples that the clinician can adapt to meet the specific needs of the population being served. The procedures listed, therefore, are not a complete taxonomy of those we have used over the years but a selected set we have found to be the most useful. Generally, individual adaptations of these procedures are required each time they are used with a child.

Chapter 6 addresses the use of elicited imitation as an assessment methodology. Major issues in using and interpreting this procedure are discussed, and several lists of sentences are included. These sentences are representative of those we use clinically to explore children's sentence imitation ability, particularly as it relates to the child's memory and information-processing ability.

The procedures in this section are included to supplement the data gathered in free-speech sample analyses where frequencies are low or specific elements require explanations. Section II, then, is a companion to Section I. Elicitation is not a substitute for free-speech analysis for documenting productive language performance.

CHAPTER 5

Elicited Production

Contents

The use of elicited production procedures is warranted when specific aspects of language are to be analyzed, when frequency of occurrence in naturalistic settings is limited, or if the usual situations do not afford detailed analysis of a specific language behavior. Where time is a factor these procedures can be quite productive in eliciting the behaviors required in a short period of time. In general, these procedures involve constructing situations in which the child is likely to emit the desired behavior. We have used specific situations to elicit questions, negative sentences, locatives, and answers to questions. In addition, procedures to elicit specific language functions—describing ongoing events, giving information, requesting information, problem solving—have been constructed for individual children.

Basic to the development of elicitation procedures is the identification of specific contexts that prompt the child to produce the behavior under study. Such contexts are different for children at different levels of cognitive development. With children younger than 3½ years of age, situations derived from the child's own experience have proved most productive, particularly those limited by discourse or formal linguistic constraints. Answers to questions, for example, either as requests for action or information, are especially productive. Consideration needs to be given to the situational constraints imposed by the linguistic dimension of interest. For example, the elicitation of negatives may be difficult when the clinical situation requires the child to be positive and compliant. Social conventions such as "Respect your elders" and "Obey adults in authority positions" may preclude responding in what we, as clinicians, would consider an optimal elicitation context.

When a specific context is identified we must ask, what does the child need to understand to perform as expected? In particular, pragmatic constraints must be identified in order to properly interpret the child's performance, especially, failures to perform as expected. For example, in the puppet show procedure to elicit Wh-questions, the child must recognize the examiner's implicit request that his or her role is to ask the puppet for the information stated by the examiner. Failures to respond appropriately can result from the child's inability to understand the pragmatic requirements of the task, either because they are not made clear in the instructions through practice and modeling or because the child exhibits pragmatic deficits in assuming another speaker's role or in identifying the appropriate circumstances for requesting information. Only if the child clearly understands the task and gives evidence of conforming to the pragmatic requirements can responses be scored for linguistic context.

INTERPRETATION OF ELICITED RESPONSES

The procedures listed in this chapter are experimental with no accompanying normative data. Given that the procedures used to elicit specific structures, meanings, or intentions only increase frequency of specific elements without constraining the child's performance in ways not associated with free-speech samples, the data from free-speech sample analyses can be used. Considerable caution should be exercised so as not to underinterpret performance where the child fails to respond or responds inappropriately due to task difficulty, novel situations, or pragmatic complexity. As well, responses can be overestimates of spontaneous speech performance if forms are modeled, allowing for imitative responses, if too few linguistic context samples are used, as with locatives and questions, or if semantic contexts are not varied, using a limited verb or noun set in eliciting inflections.

These procedures are best interpreted as estimates of spontaneous performances to be compared with free-speech samples where possible. In addition, they can be used to monitor changes in a child's performance over time when developmental status is not of immediate concern.

When constructed appropriately, elicited production procedures can increase the efficiency and specificity of assessing language behaviors that occur infrequently in natural language. The procedures listed in this chapter are particularly appropriate for children between 3½ and 12 years of age.

These procedures can be used as presented or can be adapted to specific children or situations. They can also serve as models for the development of new procedures to elicit a variety of constructions not presented in this chapter. It is important to keep in mind that respondent behavior of the child is the goal, not the procedure itself. A number of procedures can be developed to elicit the same behavior; therefore, the more simple and direct the procedure for elicitation the better. Procedural complexity does not lead to increased measurement specificity.

ELICITING Wh-QUESTIONS: PUPPET SHOW PROCEDURE

Shelly Werner, Carol C. Goossens, and Ellen E. Green

Age: 3–6 years

Purpose: To assess syntactic-semantic expression of Wh-questions

Materials: Puppet booth, Clarence the Clown puppet, suitcase, clothes, chest of drawers

Procedure: The child is watching a puppet show. Clinician introduces situation with the following narrative:

"This is my friend Clarence the Clown. He loves questions. To make him talk we have to ask him questions. Let's make Clarence talk."

The clinician then models various questions each eliciting a response from Clarence. During the procedure, the child will be given approximately 3 seconds to produce a question spontaneously. If there is no spontaneous production, the clinician cues the child by using an indirect form, i.e., "I wonder why Clarence is mad." (See Table 1 for an example.)

Scoring: Syntactically appropriate/inappropriate. See Chapter 2, Table 14 for a description of Wh-question development. Note Wh-word used as well as form.

An interactive variation of the puppet show procedure can be set up as follows:

Purpose: To assess syntactic-semantic expression of Wh-questions.

Materials: Stimulus pictures, in color, set up in an easel-like manner.

Procedure: The child and the clinician take turns asking each other Wh-questions in response to pictorial stimuli. Demonstration items are employed so the procedure can be modeled for the child. Stimulus pictures are chosen so they are paired according to semantic relations. When the child asks a question, the clinician gives a wrong answer or says "I don't know." In this way the examiner is able to determine if the child understands the semantic notion of the Wh-word used.

Example:

Clinician looks at first picture in a pair and asks, "Who is cooking?" (Child responds).

Child looks at next picture pair and asks, "Who is painting?" (Examiner responds incorrectly and child corrects).

Scoring:
1. Correct/incorrect—semantics analyzed
2. Note syntax used.

Table 1. Example of the puppet show procedure

Situation	Examiner's Cue	Child's Question	Semantic Relation	Puppet's Response
Clarence is angrily pulling his clothes out of his chest of drawers, stuffing them into a suitcase.	I wonder what Clarence is doing?	*What* are you doing?	Action	I'm packing
Clarence continues to pack.	I wonder why Clarence is packing?	*Why* are you packing?	Causality	I'm mad at George: Oh did he make me mad.
Clarence paces up and down the floor muttering to himself.	I wonder who George is?	*Who* is George?	Person	George is a clown, too. He lives downstairs (looks down). You cut that out, George.
	I wonder why Clarence is mad at George?	*Why* are you mad?	Causality	Do you know what that George did? He kicked *my* dog.

MODELING PROCEDURE FOR ELICITING Wh-QUESTIONS

Susan Marks, Helene Frye-Osler, Joe Reichle, and Shelley Schwimmer-Gluck

Age: 3–6 years

Purpose: To assess the child's use of question types in non-imitative task.

Materials: Blocks, dollhouse, toy mommy, toy daddy, ball, dog, car, shoe, bed, blanket, and boat

Procedure: Questions are elicited by having the clinician act out stories or set up tasks that require a question from the child in order for the task to be completed. Stories and tasks are arranged such that there are four separate levels of elicitation.

Fill-in-the-slot Examiner tells child a story about toy items.

e.g., "Here's a doggie. Here's a daddy. Doggie runs away. Daddy asks ____________." (Child fills in question.)

If this technique elicits no question, the clinician gives the answer and moves on to the next item.

Deferred imitation All items inappropriately responded to in fill in the slot are repeated. If the child responds appropriately, he or she is scored as successfully answering questions in a *deferred task* (upon a failure in fill-in-the-slot, the answer is given). If the child still fails to correctly respond, a direct imitation paradigm is implemented. Good performance in deferred imitations suggests environmental modeling techniques may be useful if intervention is indicated.

Direct imitation The examiner immediately provides the appropriate answer and repeats the trial on the spot. If the child responds, he or she is credited with *direct imitation* indicating a good prognosis for an imitative training paradigm.

No overt cue This class is best defined by example. The clinician places a clicker under the table and without the child's knowledge makes clicking sound and waits for the child to produce "What is it?". (Also see items #1, #3, #7 in Table 2). This technique can be integrated within a free-speech session to attempt to increase question frequency.

Table 2. Sample Contexts For Eliciting *Wh*-Questions

	Answer Sheet		
	Level of Correct Response	Child's Production	Analysis (Bellugi-Klima, 1968)
Overt Verbal Cue, Fill in the Slot			
1. "Here's doggie. Here's the Daddy. Doggie runs away, all gone. Daddy asks, '__________?' " Elicits: Where is it? (Location)	(Note: adequate room should be appropriated so child's utterance and analysis can be done.)		
2. "Daddy's driving the car. He's going someplace. Mommy asks, '__________?' " Elicits: *Where are you going? (Direction)*			
3. "Daddy finds a toy. It's not Daddy's. It's not Mommy's. Daddy asks, '__________?' " Elicits: *Whose is it?* (Possession)			
4. "Daddy hears someone in the kitchen. It's not Mommy. It's not Doggie. Daddy asks, '________?' " Elicits: *Who is it?* (Person)			
No Overt Cue, Verbal Instruction			
5. "Here's a key." (Clinician hides it under two cloths, but keeps in hand.) Elicits: Where is it? (Location)			
6. (Half hidden toy animal under cloth.) Clinician says, "It's not a cat. It's not a doggie." Elicits: *What is it?*(Object)			
7. "There are pennies. There's one for me. I don't know if there are enough." Elicits: *How many?* (Quantity)			
8. "There's candy. I have one. There's one for Mommy, I don't know if there are enough." Elicits: *How many?* (Quantity)[a]			
9. (Clinician places dog under blanket. Moves blanket to suggest doggie is doing something.) "Here's doggie. He's not running. He's not barking." Elicits: *What is he doing?* (Action)			
10. (Candy presented) "It's not mine. . . . . It's not yours." Elicits: *Whose is it?* (Possession)			
11. "There's someone under here." (Clinician moves finger under cloth to signify movement.) Elicits: *Who's that?* (Person)			
No Overt Cue, Nonverbal Instruction			
12. (Clinician hides M&M in hand. Show to child. Drops candy out of sight.) Elicits: *Where is it?* (Location)			
13. (Clinician manipulates a toy clicker that is out of sight.) Elicits: *What is that?* (Object)			
14. (Clinician pretends to toss a make believe object in bag. Makes noise with bag to suggest object was thrown in bag.) Elicits: *What's that?* (Object)			

Statements in quotation marks are those said by examiner. Statements in parenthesis are actions performed by examiner.
[a]Child may not know concept "enough," if so drop to deferred imitation.

BELLUGI'S INTERROGATION TEST[1]

Concentrate on eliciting questions that are structurally difficult or infrequent. Using dolls or puppets, tell the child to "Ask the doll ____________," using the indirect form of the question (e.g., "Ask the doll what she wants"). The verb phrase can be anything appropriate to the situation.

For example:

Vary interrogative word
- What she wants
- Where she put it
- When she'll do it
- How she got it

Vary noun phrase and auxiliary verb
- What she can do
- What I might have
- What they will have been doing
- What the boy is supposed to see

Vary with negative
- Why she doesn't help
- Why he won't come out now
- Why I can't do it
- Why they aren't here yet

Vary subject and object
- Who pushed John
- Who did John push

This procedure can be modified for older children by bringing a stranger into the room and, through the list of prompts given above, directing the child to find out who it is, and why the stranger is there.

---

[1]See Slobin (1967) for a complete explanation of Bellugi's Interrogation Test.

BELLUGI'S TAG QUESTION TEST[2]

Children begin to produce tag questions ("He is here, isn't he?") relatively late in their grammatical development. The tag question follows a statement, and generally asks for confirmation of the statement. The same purpose could be served by less elegant means: "He's here, right?", "You have some candies, huh?" or "Okay?" Children use the less elegant constructions for some time before they begin to produce tag questions.

Tag questions are particularly interesting because the shape of the tag is explicitly determined by the syntax of the statement it follows. In words, tag formation involves the following processes:

1. Pronominalize the noun phrase subject of the sentence.
2. Locate (and perhaps supply *do* or the full form of) the first auxiliary verb of the main clause of the sentence.
3. Negate the auxiliary of the sentence if affirmative. Do not negate if the sentence is negative.
4. Invert the auxiliary verb and the pronominalized noun phrase.

When children begin using tags, they do not produce tags frequently, and neither children nor adults produce the full range of possibilities in spontaneous speech. Since each tag is determined by the sentence, we can elicit tag questions from children and adults. In this way, we can gain a good deal of information about children's ability to locate the subject of a sentence, pronominalize nouns and noun phrases, handle conjoined noun phrases, define sentence negation, handle auxiliaries that they may not produce, locate the first element of an auxiliary verb, handle subject-verb agreement and tense agreement, define the subject and auxiliary of an imperative sentence, and so forth.

One could begin eliciting tag questions using a set of instructions like the following:

> Suppose I want to say something, and I'm not really sure about it. I might say: "The sun is shining today," and then, I might add; "Isn't it?" We're going to play a game like that. I'll say something, and you add the last part, like this. I say, "That alligator can bite very hard," and you say "________________."

Examples of the range of information available in tag questions are suggested in Table 3. The verb phrase part of the sentence may be varied to anything appropriate to the situation.

---

[2]See Slobin (1967) for a complete explanation of Bellugi's Tag Question Test.

Table 3. Examples of the range of information available in tag questions (Bellugi, in Slobin, 1967)

Affirmative/negative interaction

I will do it.
I won't do it.

He could come.
He couldn't come.

Be* and *have

It's been done now.
It's coming now.

John's tired.
John's finished his lunch.

They're doing it.
I was going.
They were annoyed.
I'm coming.

First element of auxiliary

He could have done it.
I will have been swimming since this morning.
They would have been coming anyway.

Tense agreement

I go there often.
I went there yesterday.

He walked farther.
He walks frequently.

Location of grammatical subject

The girl pushed the boy.
The boy was pushed by the girl.
John and you played together.
Three boys and a girl are playing together.

Definition of sentence negation

He came here.
He never came.

He is unhappy.
He is happy.

I saw the boy who didn't go to school.
The boy who didn't go to school was fishing.

Nobody likes me.
Everybody likes me.

They have no sense.
They have little sense.

Modal auxiliaries

I could have found it.
They should arrive soon.
He will ask us.
She can do it.

Subject and auxiliary of imperatives

Help me find this book.
Sit down.
Come here.

***Do* as auxiliary verb**

I need some cookies.
You see the truck.

Subject-verb agreement

I hit the ball.
He hits the ball.

You throw the stone.
John throws the stone.

Pronominalization

John came home early.
Sue is running.
The boys are playing.
The chair tipped over.

Both of them did it.
The two of us want some.

John and Bill played together.
John and I played together.

Yesterday after we came home from a long walk, the little girl came out to greet us.
I know where the boy is hiding.
The boys who jumped over the fence in my neighbors' yard ran away.

Limit on applicability of tag

Who finished this?

ELICITING NEGATIVE STRUCTURES THROUGH ROLE-PLAYING

Susan Schmidt

The procedures that have been developed to elicit particular linguistic structures seem to be more appropriate for the older child. By examining the nature of an elicitation task we might be able to hypothesize why. Bellugi (1967) has suggested a procedure to elicit negation. The task is described as such: The child is asked to provide the negative of a sentence spoken by the investigator. The instruction given to the child is: "I'll say something and then you say the opposite. I'll say *You can see him* and you say *You can't see him.*" A list of sentences is then presented to the child. This task is confounded by the use of the concept "opposite." If the child has no understanding of that particular concept he or she will not be able to perform the task. Also, this procedure is based on the exchange of verbatim information with little or no context to aid the younger child. If a procedure to elicit negation provided more contextual clues for the child would it be more appropriate for the preschooler?

While observing prekindergarten children as they played, it was noticed that many children were involved in role-playing games. Parten (1933) watched the play of 34 nursery schoolers and obtained 60 behavioral samples on each child. She reported that sandbox play was by far the most preferred and playing make-believe games, such as "family," "house," or "dolls," was second. There were group trends toward an increased amount of make-believe play with increasing age for the 3- to 4-year-old children (Singer, 1973). This ability to role-play could possibly be tapped as a technique in assessment of the young child. The role that the child is to play should be one that is familiar to the child. The subjects in this assessment procedure are asked to play the role of a mother.

This task makes use of role-playing as an assessment technique to elicit negative structures from the child.

Materials and Setting: A small room equipped with two tables, a counter, a blackboard, a set of dishes, empty food cartons, plastic food, and a makeshift stove. The list of structures to be tested should be written on the blackboard as an aid to the examiner. Tape record the session for later transcription and analysis (see Table 4 for sample format).

Procedure: The child is brought into the room and told that she and the examiner are going to play a game. The following instructions are given: "You're the mommy and I'm your little girl. I did something really bad this morning and you're *mad* at me. So everything I say or anything I want to do, you say I can't do it 'cause you're *mad* at me. So if I say 'Mommy, can I watch TV?', you say, 'No you can't watch TV.'" A few more models are presented and then the game starts. No structure is placed on the activity, the examiner follows the mother's (subject's) lead and when appropriate asks the test items. Both subjects end up making the examiner's breakfast.

During the activity the examiner presents various items that the child is to negate. These items vary in their construction. The verb tenses vary, modals "can" and "may" can be introduced, and the indefinite pronouns "somebody" and "someone" used. See Table 4 for sample prompts and responses from two children. Whenever a test item is being asked, the examiner deliberately varies the intonation shift, which provides a cue to the child that he or she is to negate that item. If the child only responds with "No," the examiner can probe further by saying "No, what?" This usually prompts the child to expand the utterance, but not in every case.

Table 4. Eliciting negative structures, sample prompts, and responses from two children

Prompts	Child #1 Age-4;6, MLU, 4.2	Child #2 Age-4;0, MLU,4.0
Modal "can"		
I can go outside.	No, you can't.	No, you can't go with Jimmy.
Can I have a cookie?	We don't have any cookies.	Nope, you can't have any.
Present progressive		
I am going to watch TV.	No. (would not expand)	No, you not gonna watch TV.
I am going outside now.		No, you not.
I am going to play with Johnny this afternoon.	No, you can't.	
Future tense		
We will go to the store today.	No, we not go to the store today.	No, we cannot.
Will you let me go outside?	No, it's too cold.	No, you can't go outside.
"Don't" construction		
Do I get to eat the candy?	No. (would not expand)	No, you can't.
My dolly likes candy.		No, she doesn't like it.
My dolly wants a cookie.	No, she can't have a cookie.	No, she can't have a cookie.
Modal "may"		
May I watch TV?	No, you can't.	No, you cannot.
May I go outside?		
Negative with indefinite		
I want some candy.	No, you can't.	No, you can't have some candy.
My dolly wants some candy.		She can't have no candy.
Someone is at the door.	Nobody at the door.	Don't let them in.
Somebody is at the door.	Nobody at the door.	Don't let them in.

Child #2 used construction spontaneously: "I won't be mad, if you behave; I won't be mad."

BELLUGI'S NEGATION TEST[1]

The child is asked to provide the negative of a sentence spoken by the investigator. The following instructions are given: "I'll say something and then you say the (opposite or negative). I'll say, *You can see him,* and you say, *You can't see him.*" Model sentences such as the following can be used:

Vary auxiliary

The dog can bark.	The dog ______.
The doll will break.	The doll ______.
The baby is crying.	The baby ______.
The boy wants a cookie.	The boy ______.
He went outside.	He ______.

Negative with indefinite (increase in complexity)

The girl ate some soup.	______.
She wants some dinner.	______.
Someone saw him.	______.
Somebody is coming in.	______.
The girl asked someone.	______.

Imperatives

Sit down there.	______.
Come at five o'clock.	______.

Multi-propositional sentences

I saw the boy who came here.	______.
He asked her to do it.	______.
Someone wants him to take some.	______.
Why does he do it?	______.

It would be valuable to first elicit imitations of the sentences from the child. This will give a clue as to what patterns are beyond the child.

The following techniques may facilitate the application of such procedures to very young subjects. The investigator should use a doll and a collection of objects. The doll should be named, perhaps by the child. The doll is then included in the test; for example: "Joe (child's name), you have a ball. Does Andy (doll's name) have a ball? Andy doesn't have a ball." The experimenter should then keep repeating, "Joe has a ball. Andy doesn't have a ball," until the child can be brought to imitate the last sentence. The test can then continue, perhaps testing another auxiliary: "Joe can run. Andy can't run." And so forth. (It might be necessary to use some reward for the imitation, like giving the child beads.)

After a run of this sort, it may be possible to offer the affirmative sentences and let the child provide the negative sentences without prompting. Perhaps the child can be encouraged to talk about "Andy."

---

[1]See Slobin (1967) for a complete explanation of Bellugi's Negation Test.

BELLUGI'S REFLEXIVIZATION TEST[4]

Reflexivization can be thought of as a grammatical process that can be elicited in a limited way. In English, when the subject and the object of certain verbs are the same, the object is reflexivized. In children's speech, one may find intermediate stages like: "I made me a telescope" or "I see me." One does not reflexivize in order to make it clear that two different people are referred to by the same pronoun. Compare: "He sees himself" and "He sees him" (another person). One can elicit, after providing one (or perhaps more) models of reflexivization. For example, suppose you have two pictures. In one, a boy is washing a dog, and in another the same boy is washing his own face. You label them: "The boy washes the dog." "The boy washes himself." On a new set of pictures the child should be asked to supply the reflexivized form. To test for comprehension of reflexivization at an earlier stage, one might use the set suggested above; that is, a boy looking at another boy; a boy looking at himself in a mirror, and ask the child to choose the appropriate picture.

If you can begin to elicit reflexives, you may use sentences to be filled in like the following:

Pronominalization

The boy washed ______________________.
The girl dressed ______________________.
The boy and the girl looked at ______________.
I see ______________________________.

Imperatives

Behave ______________________________.
Protect ______________________________.

Sentence boundary A particular rule in English is that reflexivization does not take place outside of sentence boundaries. That is, we reflexivize propositions. Thus, in these sentences, one cannot reflexivize the subject of the main clause.

I want her to take care of ____________. (Not myself)
John wanted Mary to help __________. (Not himself)

[4]See Slobin (1967) for a complete explanation of Bellugi's Reflexivization Test.

WORD ORDER IN PRODUCTION: AN ELICITATION TASK

Robin S. Chapman and Jon F. Miller (1975)

Ages: 20–32 months

Purpose: This procedure is designed to elicit from the child sentences depending states of affairs in which subject and object roles were varied. With this procedure the child's use of word order in sentence production can be observed in controlled contexts to determine its consistency.

Materials: Plain wooden car, a dump truck, a sailboat, flexible boy and girl dolls, and a plastic dog. Objects should be of similar size.

Procedure: The child watches the experimenter perform an action with two of the six toys and is asked to describe the action in a sentence through one of the following instructions, whichever proves most effective: "What's happening?" "What's going on?" "What am I doing?" The task is preceded by sample sentences in which the experimenter models the child's response, if necessary. If the child becomes inattentive, the experimenter demonstrates the action and then allows the child to demonstrate it while producing a description.

Pretesting: To ensure that the child knows the lexical items used in constructing the sentences, each item is pretested by asking the child to point to each toy as it is named. The child is then asked to name each toy as the experimenter points to it. The actions exemplified by each of the six verbs are then labeled and demonstrated to the child. For instance, the experimenter would say, "hitting," while demonstrating *boy hitting girl.* The child is then asked to demonstrate and produce each of the six verbs following their production and demonstration by the experimenter. (See Table 5.) Responses to the production task are scored specifically for the appropriate ordering of the subject and object with respect to the verb. The categories used are *correct,* including subject-verb-object, subject-verb, verb-object, or subject-object sentences (synonym substitutions are accepted); *wrong,* including object-verb-subject, verb-subject, object-verb, or object-subject sentences; *no response;* or undecidable, including all responses on which subject-object ordering cannot be determined (for example, verb only). The guessing rate for correctly ordering subject, object, or both subject and object with respect to the verb in a scorable response would be 50% following these scoring procedures.

Table 5. Sample sentences for word order task

Subject, Object	Original sentences	Subject, Object	Reversed versions
+ Animate + Animate	The boy is hitting the girl. The girl is carrying the dog. The dog is chasing the boy.	+ Animate + Animate	The girl is hitting the boy. The dog is carrying the girl. The boy is chasing the dog.
+ Animate – Animate	The dog is chasing the car. The boy is carrying the truck. The girl is pulling the boat.	– Animate + Animate	The car is chasing the dog. The truck is carrying the boy. The boat is pulling the girl.
– Animate + Animate	The boat is hitting the girl. The truck is bumping the dog. The car is pushing the boy.	+ Animate – Animate	The girl is hitting the boat. The dog is bumping the truck. The boy is pushing the car.
– Animate – Animate	The truck is pulling the boat. The boat is bumping the car. The car is pushing the truck.	– Animate – Animate	The boat is pulling the truck. The car is bumping the boat. The truck is pushing the car.

CHAPTER 6

Elicited Imitation

In elicited imitation tasks, the child is required to repeat a list of stimulus sentences read by the examiner. Usually, sentence lists consist of sentence sets that vary in grammatical form. In using elicited imitation tasks in assessment, the clinician must make the following assumptions:

1. Linguistic processing occurs in repetition tasks.
2. Repetition tasks involve short-term memory processes.
3. Sentence processing in short-term memory is dependent upon the linguistic knowledge available to the child.
4. If stimulus sentences exceed the child's short-term memory span, then the child must rely upon his or her linguistic knowledge to facilitate memory in order to correctly repeat the sentence.
5. Since the child's knowledge of the language provides an organizational strategy for short-term memory in processing incoming linguistic stimuli, his or her imitative responses should index his or her knowledge of the language, particularly the structural or grammatical components.

A careful review of the elicited imitation literature reveals that these assumptions are not always justified. The results of many studies are conflicting and do not allow a clear interpretation of exactly what linguistic elements are processed: structural, semantic, or both. Several studies conclude that language processing does not occur in elicited imitation (Fraser, Bellugi, and Brown, 1963; Lovell and Dixon, 1965; DeArmengol, Goldstein, and Lombana, 1974). Other studies assume elicited imitation allows inferences to be drawn about children's syntactic production system (Menyuk, 1963; Lackner, 1968; Smith, 1970; Slobin and Welsh, 1973; Carrow, 1974; Kuczaj and Maratsos, 1975). Several studies conclude that elicited imitative responses do reveal some information about comprehension or production of syntax (Menyuk, 1969; Smith, 1970; Slobin and Welsh, 1973; Kuczaj and Maratsos, 1975).

It is generally agreed that some processing takes place in elicited imitation procedures. However, it is not clear what is processed or whether this processing is related to comprehension processes or production processes. In addition, a number of variables affect performance: context (Bloom, 1974), sentence length (Miller, 1973; Miller and Chapman, 1975), and scoring (Miller and Yoder, 1973). The appropriate interpretation of children's responses on elicited imitation tasks remains unclear (Hood and Lightbown, 1978). We have found, however, that these tasks are useful in certain situations. They should never be the only procedure administered to determine level of syntactic performance. When used in conjunction with direct measures of comprehension and production, they can provide useful information about: 1) the child's ability to process sentences auditorily in the absence of context; 2) the child's memory ability for sentences; 3) the relationship among imitation, comprehension, and production abilities of the child that is necessary in determining treatment strategies—many children cannot imitate sentences they are capable of comprehending (Miller and Yoder, 1973); and 4) the presence or absence of auditory processing problems.

Although elicited imitation procedures are easy to use, it is not clear at this time what responses on these tasks mean clinically. Additionally, assumptions derived from normal populations may not apply to deviant populations, since deviant populations evidence different memory processes, as in retarded children, and other processing difficulties that complicate our ability to infer knowledge from imitative responses.

In developing sentence sets for use with elicited imitation tasks several factors must be controlled if we are to compare performance across sentences. The sample sentence set in Table 1 is taken from the Miller-Yoder Test of Grammatical Comprehension (in preparation). These sentences were constructed to be as similar to each other as possible except for grammatical form. Specific attention was paid to:

1. *Sentence Length* Most sentences are five words in length.
2. *Semantic Complexity* Most sentences express a single underlying proposition.
3. *Vocabulary* The vocabulary for the entire sentence set is as small as possible, with complexity minimized.

Children's performance on this sentence set can not only be compared directly with their comprehension of the same sentences but imitation performance can be compared across grammatical form because length, complexity, and vocabulary have been controlled. Another strategy for developing sentence sets to compare with spontaneous production is to use the developmental data in the ASS tables for simple sentences and the complex sentence analysis, both in Chapter 2. These tables, along with the child's transcript, provide the target forms both within and beyond the child's level of development. Using the child's own expressed vocabulary, sentence sets can be developed to test directly the child's ability to imitate sentences containing forms within his or her repertoire and those not yet acquired. By further varying sentence length as well, the relative contribution of memory versus grammatical complexity can be evaluated.

Interpretations of imitation performance must be made by inference. Imitation assesses neither comprehension or production directly. However, imitation tasks are valuable clinical devices in solving problems of children's performance when stimuli are controlled properly. Review the sentence set in the same transcription format below. Given that 5-year-old normal children would be able to repeat exactly these five-word sentences 90% of the time, how would you make them more difficult? *In clinical practice we must develop more of our own materials lest we approach language as a routine set of surface forms rather than rule-governed, creative and representational, transcending time and space.*

SUGGESTED TRANSCRIPTION FORMAT

1. List stimulus sentences in the order they are to be administered with sufficient spacing to allow notations to be made.
2. Tape-record the testing session.
3. Using the list of stimulus sentences as a guide, cross out elements not imitated by the child, add elements expressed that were not part of the stimulus sentence, and indicate phrases. If phonetic or phonological information is required, the initial list should be phonetic rather than orthographic to facilitate accurate stimulus presentation and to provide a model for recording the child's responses. See sample format on opposite page.

~~THE~~ PENCIL ~~IS~~ GREEN

~~THE~~ LITTLE BOY ~~IS~~ EATING SOME PINK ICE CREAM

~~THE~~ OWL EATS CANDY ~~AND~~ RUNS FAST

~~THE~~ BOY THE BOOK ~~HIT~~ WAS CRYING

WHAT WILL HE SING?

I SAW THE MAN ~~AND~~ ~~THE~~ MAN ATE THE ICE CREAM

Table 1. Sample sentence set from Miller-Yoder Test of Grammatical Comprehension (Miller and Yoder, in preparation)

A. **Active Subject/Object**
1. The boy washes the girl.
   The girl washes the boy.
2. The cat chases the dog.
   The dog chases the cat.

B. **Preposition**
on/under
3. John sits on the table.
   John sits under the table.
4. Spot stands on the bed.
   Spot stands under the bed.

in/beside
5. Sally stands in the box.
   Sally stands beside the box.
6. John sits in the tree.
   John sits beside the tree.

C. **Possessive**
7. Show me the boy's daddy.
   Show me the daddy's boy.
8. Show me the girl's mother.
   Show me the mother's girl.

D. **Negative/Affirmative Statements**
has/doesn't have
9. John has a hat.
   John doesn't have a hat.
10. Sally has a dress.
    Sally doesn't have a dress.

can/can't
11. John can catch the ball.
    John can't catch the ball.
12. John can carry the box.
    John can't carry the box.

is/is not
13. The dog is running.
    The dog is not running.
14. The man is working.
    The man is not working.

E. **Pronouns**
Object
her/them
15. John is riding with her.
    John is riding with them.

him/her
16. Spot is barking at her.
    Spot is barking at him.

him/them
17. Sally is walking with him.
    Sally is walking with them.

Subject
he/they
18. He splashes the girl.
    They splash the girl.

she/they
19. They eat the cookies.
    She eats the cookies.

he/she
20. He is making a picture.
    She is making a picture.

subject/object

21. He is yelling at her.
    She is yelling at him.
22. He jumps over them.
    They jump over him.
23. She hides from them.
    They hide from her.

F. **Singular/Plural**

Noun

24. Show me the marbles.
    Show me the marble.
25. Show me the blocks.
    Show me the block.

Noun/Verb Inflections

26. The cat climbs the tree.
    The cats climb the tree.
27. The boy rides the horse.
    The boys ride the horse.

Verb (is/are)

28. The sheep is eating.
    The sheep are eating.
29. The deer is jumping.
    The deer are jumping.

G. Verb Inflections

Present Progressive/Future

30. John is building a house.
    John will build a house.

Present Progressive/Past

31. Sally is sewing the dress.
    Sally sewed the dress.

Future/Past

32. Spot will bury the bone.
    Spot buried the bone.

H. **Modification**

Object

33. John has a little truck.
    John has a big truck.
34. Sally has a red ball.
    Sally has a green ball.

Subject

35. The little dog is sleeping.
    The big dog is sleeping.
36. The blue bird is flying.
    The black bird is flying.

Subject/Object

37. Red birds eat big berries.
    Blue birds eat little berries.
38. Big boys have round blocks.
    Little boys have square blocks.

I. **Reversible Passives**

39. John is pushed by Sally.
    Sally is pushed by John.
40. Mother is kissed by father.
    Father is kissed by mother.

J. **Reflexivization**

41. The girl is feeding her.
    The girl is feeding herself.
42. The boy is squirting him.
    The boy is squirting himself.

SECTION III

INTEGRATING ASSESSMENT DATA

CHAPTER 7

Interpretation

Contents

While the focus of this volume is the assessment of children's productive language, data from other processes are necessary for interpretation. As discussed in previous work (Miller, 1978), not just production but language comprehension and cognitive development must be evaluated to establish a child's language performance (see Table 1). Each of these developmental processes is multidimensional and provides a number of data points that must be coordinated in developing a framework for interpreting an individual child's performance status.

Basic to the interpretation of production data is a reminder that the selection of approaches and analysis procedures for individual children is of primary importance. The meaning of assessment data is dependent upon the validity of the procedures and the analysis chosen. Given the variety of processes and linguistic domains affected in children with suspect language performance, procedures must be selected individually for each child. Decisions regarding choice of assessment procedures for each child require consideration of a number of variables before the evaluation. The development of an evaluation plan is basic to deriving the language performance data that is to be interpreted.

This planning process does not presume assessment to be a one time affair conducted before the initiation of intervention. The planning process is essential in selecting valid measures of child performance. Assessment is a continual process of asking

Table 1. Developmental processes and performance dimensions necessary for interpreting language performance status

Processes	Performance dimensions assessed
Cognitive development	*Nonstandard measures* of nonverbal mental abilities such as those described in Piaget's developmental psychology *Psychometric description* Mental age determined by standardized measures of nonverbal (performance) mental abilities.
Comprehension	Lexicon, syntax-semantics, pragmatics
Production	Phonology, syntax, semantics, pragmatics

questions, deciding which procedures can answer them, collecting assessment data, and interpreting the data to determine language performance status. This process invariably results in the emergence of a new set of questions requiring further evaluation.

DEVELOPING AN EVALUATION PLAN[1]

In developing formats for evaluation with specific goals, it is important to remember that children whose language behavior is questionable in terms of development and use are found in a number of different settings and programs. Each service program has its own unique purpose, characteristics, and goals relative to the educational, habilitative, or rehabilitative services provided for the specific population(s) served. That individual educational and clinical service facilities differ implies that evaluation formats will vary as well. Although basic communication processes are evaluated in every case, assessment formats should be individualized for each setting according to the following three basic principles:

1. Evaluations should be consistent with the purpose and goals of the individual service program in terms of breadth, depth, and objectives.
2. Evaluation formats or decision-making plans should be constructed for each type of evaluation performed.
3. Any evaluation of communication behavior must be responsive to individual variation in etiology and the general developmental level of the child.

These three principles point out that individual assessment formats will differ depending upon the type of program or service setting in which the evaluation occurs, the goal of evaluation performed, and the individual characteristics of the child to be evaluated. A screening performed in an elementary school setting differs from a baseline evaluation performed in a diagnostic clinic in terms of: 1) goal—problem identification versus developmental level of language use, 2) breadth and depth—school-related curricular issues versus language use in communicating a variety of intentions and topics and minimally detailed versus extensively detailed program planning, and 3) population—minimally involved, essentially normal versus developmentally delayed and multiply handicapped children. The interaction of setting, goal, and population in developing individual assessment formats points out the complexities the clinician faces in attempting to evaluate children's communication behavior.

Our overall evaluation objectives are to individualize a developmental assessment format for each child that reflects service program objectives, evaluation goals, and specific populations served. These objectives point out the need for a flexible decision-making framework that is hierarchical and is adaptable to different situations and goals.

The approach we have used in the development of an individualized decision-making system is the basic scientific method. Its application requires a basic understanding of the processes to be studied: language development and use, physiological processes involved, and environmental influences. Procedurally, it can be compared to conducting a research study: explore relevant background research (reports, observations), formulate a hypothesis (determine which questions to ask), select a procedure to test the hypothesis (i.e., to answer the questions), administer the procedure, analyze the results, interpret the results with appropriate criteria, formulate conclusions, and make recommendations.

The formulation of an individualized assessment plan is essentially the planning of a research study with an *N* of one. The implementation of such a plan should lead to an objective appraisal of individual dimensions of communication behavior, which allows for the selection of a variety of procedures and subsequent questions to be asked when a more detailed analysis is required.

Let us briefly discuss the assessment format we have developed for establishing baseline functioning in an interdisciplinary clinic. The overview of the format is presented in Figure 1.

The first task is to determine the child's general level of development through reading reports of previous evaluations, referrals, etc., or by observing the child directly. With a general level of development established (the child appears to be functioning like a 2-, 3-, or 4-year-old) we have a basis from which to ask questions about his or her communication behavior. These questions will be addressed to two different sources, the child and the parent(s). The major areas in which questions should be addressed about the child's performance are shown in Figure 1. Questions may be general or specific, depending upon the amount of information available about the child. They could be as general as, "What is the child's general level of grammatical comprehension?" or as specific as, "What locatives does the child understand in the absence of context?" Unless there is sufficient information to preclude it, questions should be asked of the child in each of the seven areas

[1]This section substantially taken from Miller, 1978, pp. 306–309.

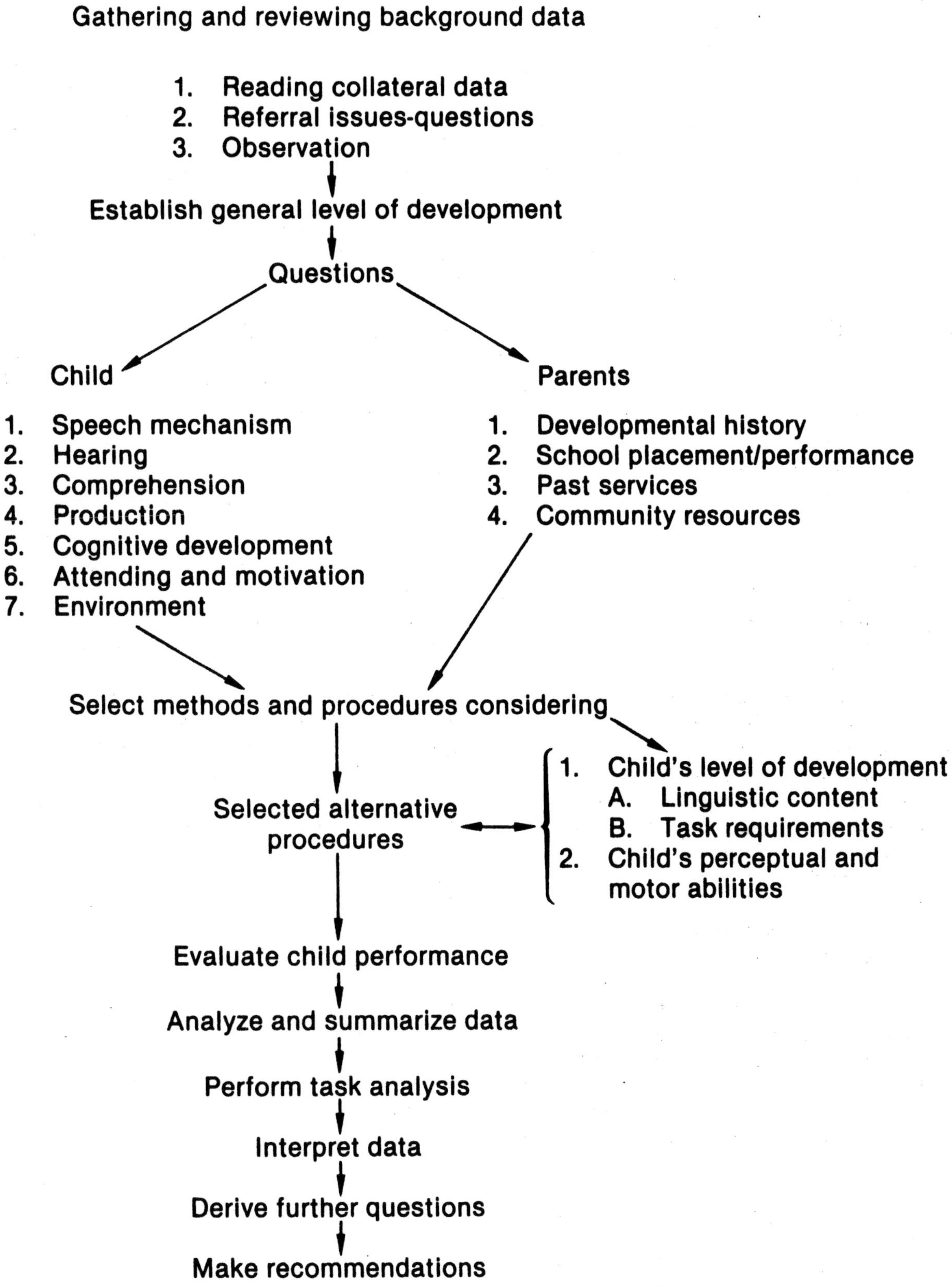

Gathering and reviewing background data

1. Reading collateral data
2. Referral issues-questions
3. Observation

Establish general level of development

Questions

Child

1. Speech mechanism
2. Hearing
3. Comprehension
4. Production
5. Cognitive development
6. Attending and motivation
7. Environment

Parents

1. Developmental history
2. School placement/performance
3. Past services
4. Community resources

Select methods and procedures considering

1. Child's level of development
   - A. Linguistic content
   - B. Task requirements
2. Child's perceptual and motor abilities

Selected alternative procedures

Evaluate child performance

Analyze and summarize data

Perform task analysis

Interpret data

Derive further questions

Make recommendations

Figure 1. Developing an evaluation plan.

listed as these represent major dimensions of language or related processes. Questions addressed to the parents may be in the three areas listed in Figure 1, although these are only sample areas. Many other questions may be used depending upon the populations served and the goals of the program.

With our questions specified, methods and procedures can be selected to answer them. The criterion for selecting a specific task or procedure is its ability to provide the information necessary to answer the question asked. Other factors affecting task selection are: the child's level of development, the linguistic content specified, the requirements the task imposes upon the child, and the child's motor and perceptual abilities. We always select alternative procedures to evaluate the same behavior, making sure the alternatives use different tasks, input modes, or motor requirements. Having alternative procedures available improves the chances of answering the assessment questions in the most efficient manner.

With tasks selected, we determine an order of presentation that will allow a variety of tasks and where possible embody several tasks in a single context. For example, in a play context, production procedures, comprehension of commands and questions, and certain cognitive tasks can be administered without changing the child's activity.

Tasks are then presented, results are analyzed and summarized, and task analyses are performed to determine if there was sufficient confounding by any of the variables that influence performance to call into question our results from specific procedures. Then we organize the results in a fashion that allows interpretation. At this point, we have sufficient information to ask further questions about specific dimensions of behavior, either to clarify our findings or to develop more specific information about the child's performance. Recommendations about treatment programs—their form, structure, and content—can be made at this point, recognizing that additional questions about the child's performance may need to be answered. These questions can be answered in the context of a treatment program and often provide the best framework for continued evaluation.

This format, then, provides for the continual interaction between assessment and treatment. Assessment should *never* be considered as a separate activity. It should always be considered a starting point in the process of decision making about each child, the initial decision being "problem/no problem." Given that the child has a significant communicative problem, evaluation should continue as an integral part of the treatment plan.

In summary, this approach to the establishment of individualized assessment formats is hierarchical. This arrangement allows questions to be asked from a general to a specific nature. It is adaptable to different situations in that the questions may be directed within each area for a specific purpose related to the mission of the setting. The format reflects the child's general abilities and developmental level, and the methods are selected specifically for that child from an array of methods that may include both standardized and nonstandardized procedures. It provides for a task analysis, as well as continuing evaluation within the context of the treatment program.

TASK ANALYSIS: A CONSIDERATION OF VARIABLES INFLUENCING PERFORMANCE

Essentially, three sets of variables affect the results of any assessment procedure: those related to the situation or place of testing, those related to the task itself, and those related to the child. The better we are able to recognize these factors and how they can potentially influence the child's language behavior the more confident we can be in interpreting our results. In discussing these variables it must be recognized that they are not independent factors but interact with one another. All of the variables are potentially operating in any one testing situation. It is imperative to evaluate aspects of the situation and the task very carefully to avoid confounding of results. Aspects of the child's behavior that may influence test results should also be noted.

Situational Variables

There are three situational variables. The first is *the setting or place of evaluation.* The general environment of the evaluation will influence the child's behavior, particularly young children. The child's familiarity and comfort in the situation appears to be the critical factor—the more familiar and comfortable the child, the more talkative the child.

The setting interacts to some extent with the second variable, *the person.* The person doing the evaluation will affect the child's responding for the same reasons the setting affects performance. An examiner who is new to the child usually will not get the same response pattern as a familiar person. In this respect, it is important, if the opportunity exists, to get to know the child before the evaluation. If no opportunity exists, then reports of behavior from

Mom, teacher, and others who know the child, or direct observation of the child interacting with a familiar person become important information sources with which to correlate the results of the clinical evaluation.

The third variable related to the setting is *the time of day,* which is of particular importance for evaluating the child in school settings. If the child is going to miss ongoing classroom activities that are enjoyed—art, movies, or recess—because of the time of the evaluation, it is likely that the child will not be very cooperative and this will influence the results. Similar situations exist in other settings. This factor also interacts with the state of the child (discussed under child variables). Time of day may affect the child's ability to respond, although this is usually more a factor with younger children (0–5 years) than older children.

Task Variables

This set of variables is most important in nonstandardized tasks, primarily because they constitute the framework for developing an adequate assessment tool. Many of these factors are controlled in standardized tests, and some consideration should be given toward evaluating all testing procedures, noting potential factors influencing the child's responses. There are seven variables related to the task.

1. Input mode Are the stimuli presented auditorily, visually, or both? Variations in children's responding should be noted relative to these different modes of input. In general, children perform better if stimuli are presented through both auditory and visual channels simultaneously than through the auditory or visual channel alone. Differential performance through auditory and visual channels will affect mode of presentation for programming.

2. Response mode Tasks may require the child to respond verbally, by manipulating objects, or by pointing to pictures. Not all children will respond equally well to these various modes of response. Also, not all children will have all response modes available to them, as with the motorically involved child. It would be self-defeating to expect such a child to manipulate objects in evaluating comprehension when a picture pointing task best fits his or her motor abilities.

3. Instructions The instructions will affect performance if they are too brief or too complex. Usually instructions are given verbally, and since this is the behavior under study, verbal instructions should be kept to a minimum with a great deal of task modeling by the clinician. Also, enough practice items should be included to make sure the task is understood by the child.

4. Stimuli The stimuli are a factor in that their careful control is essential if results are to be meaningful. In elicited imitation tasks, for example, we know that sentence length directly affects performance (Miller, 1973). If sentence stimuli vary in length and complexity, the child's responses may be a function of length rather than sentence complexity. This is a difficult, but all-important, variable to consider if our results are to be meaningful. Children with visual modality problems may have difficulty perceiving and processing pictures that represent objects or actions. An error in responding may be the result of the acuity or perceptual problems rather than lack of knowledge of a concept or word meaning.

5. Context This factor has reference to the materials the child is asked to deal with: pictures, objects, etc. In obtaining a speech sample for production analysis, objects are better stimuli than pictures because the examiner does not have to probe as much with questions. Also, new or unique toys given to the child elicit more speech than old and common ones. In elicited tasks, the objects should be appropriate to age or functioning level of the child. Failure in this regard will result in a lack of inherent motivation that the task may have for the child, with resulting lack of performance. Attending to this factor can result in increased motivation and attending by the child, save time, and increase confidence of valid and reliable results.

6. Order of Presentation This variable only affects the elicited imitation and elicited production tasks. Sentences in these tasks should be randomized for presentation to avoid having the child form a set or expectation on the sentence form or content. For example, if all negative sentences are presented together, the child may develop a particular set in responding to them that does not require processing the whole sentence. This can be avoided by randomizing the presentation of sentences.

7. Scoring Scoring has implications for the usefulness of the information gathered. The major factor to be kept in mind here is that the primary goal of assessment is to determine developmental status relative to age and cognitive level expectations. Scoring procedures should allow the summary of results in a form that leads toward this goal. It should be recognized that both numerical scores quantifying developmental status and stage descriptions of performance are necessary to document status and describe performance sufficiently in initiating intervention where appropriate.

In addition, scoring of responses on nonstandardized procedures may affect results directly. For example, with an elicited imitation task, criteria for correct response may be exact imitation of the sentence or repetition of the basic meaning elements of the sentence. The choice between these two criteria will affect the number of correct responses and therefore the interpretation of the results. The same situation exists with comprehension scoring where single sentences or sentence pairs may be used as previously discussed. For sentence pairs both must be correct before the child is credited with understanding the construction. With single sentences only a correct response on each is necessary to credit understanding. Sentence pair scoring is the more rigid criterion with fewer correct responses resulting but confidence is increased in reporting the results. See Owings (1972) for a discussion of this point relative to comprehension testing.

Child Variables

This set of variables is related to what the child brings to the task in terms of abilities and mechanisms directly related to performance on various language assessment tasks. Seven variables are listed, although there are probably others to be considered.

1. Memory Memory affects probably every language assessment task developed thus far—some in a primary way, and others less directly. For the most part, language evaluations in general seek to tap the child's linguistic knowledge held in long-term memory. Short-term memory (STM) is a primary part of the information processing system and deficits in STM must be considered when errors occur on testing procedures. For example, in comprehension testing, errors could be the result of the inability to deal with the linguistic construction presented, or the failure to hold the sentence long enough in STM to process it and make the appropriate response. STM is a primary component in imitation tasks. We have found that children with a random word memory span of less than three items could not successfully repeat five word sentences. In fact, random word memory span correlated highly (r=0.87) with the number of sentences imitated by mentally retarded children. In sentence imitation, children retrieve the syntactic structure along with marking lexical items for appropriate syntactic and semantic function, then they fill in the syntactic structure with the lexical items from the stimulus sentence remaining in STM. Memory, then, is a primary behavior related to language use.

2. Attention and Motivation Attending to the task presented is always of concern when evaluating behavior. Attending, however, should not be viewed as an independent behavior. It is directly tied to the child's motivation (variable number 3), and the two are not easily separated. Usually if the task is motivating or motivating contingencies are built in, i.e., reinforcing consequences, the child will attend to the task. Any lapses in attending while the child is completing the task are easily recognizable, and antecedent and consequent events surrounding these incidences can be described.

3. Sensory (Auditory-visual sensory system functioning) This variable is noted merely to point out the obvious. Hearing testing and vision testing should be completed when sensory system integrity is in question, before language is assessed. The perceptual processing characteristics are as important to look at as the acuity aspects.

4. Physiological Noting the child's motor development is important for task selection. Those children with limited motor ability will have obvious difficulty with tasks involving gross motor responses such as object manipulation. Such tasks, then, should obviously be avoided. Task selection should be based, in part, on the response modes available to the child.

Limited motor ability may also affect the child's interaction with the environment, thus potentially affecting a necessary component in early language learning.

The physiological integrity of the speech mechanism is critical for production. Every evaluation should include a speech mechanism exam to determine if the child has the necessary structures and functional abilities required for the production of speech. It is not possible to evaluate linguistic production in the absence of a viable speech mechanism.

5. Experiential History The child's history of involvement with the environment, both linguistic and nonlinguistic, is important for selecting motivating contexts, selecting lexical items for use in sentences for imitation and elicited production tasks, and interpreting the analysis of spontaneous language samples. If the child is unfamiliar with the objects presented and the vocabulary used, or uses a dialectical variation of the community language, the evaluation results will be affected. Usually an interview with parents, regarding the child's language development and activities in which he or she is currently interested, will provide the necessary data to avoid this problem.

6. State The state of the child is of particular importance for younger children where hunger and fatigue greatly affect behavior. However, the state variable should not be overlooked in older children where certain emotional and biological states affect the evaluation results. As pointed out under situational variables, state is often directly related to time of day.

It should be recognized that in other evaluation systems some of the variables influencing performance are evaluated directly with the assumption that they are causal factors in resultant performance. These factors may indeed influence language performance, but they can only be observed in the context of evaluating language behavior directly. Such factors as input and output mode, memory, attention, motivation, and state of the child are influenced by the task and content. They cannot, therefore, be evaluated independently if we intend to generalize results to language performance. Judgments about the child's attention and motivation can only be made under various stimulus and reinforcement contexts with situations controlled to maximize performance. Only then can we determine if problems exist in these areas, which, of course, is essential to determination of a careful, well-motivated treatment plan.

Careful evaluation of each assessment in terms of these influencing variables constitutes a task analysis system. Clearly, it would be difficult, if not impossible, to keep all these variables in mind while interacting with a child. Our goal, however, is to use the task analysis to note potential biasing factors in the child's behavior that will affect interpretation, to improve our own evaluative skills through self-evaluation and reflection on the session, and to serve as a basis for asking further questions about the child's language behavior. At our present level of development, task analysis is a painful but necessary process if we are to improve our ability to make informed clinical judgments.

DETERMINING DEVELOPMENTAL STATUS[2]

Determining developmental status for individual children involves summarizing the data for performance dimensions assessed both within and between each developmental process. Each process assessed is developmental in nature, and a developmental level can be assigned for each dimension evaluated within individual processes (See Table 1). For example, the dimensions of the production process are the child's phonological, syntactic, semantic, and pragmatic development. Taken together, the child's development of these dimensions represents the developmental level of the production process. Each process is multidimensional, i.e., is usually comprised of several distinct dimensions, and is assumed to be hierarchical, e.g., earlier levels of development are necessary for later periods of development.

The dimensions of each process are mutually dependent in development. Achievements in phonology are necessary for lexical development, and achievements in lexical development are necessary for syntactic development. Although these dimensions are mutually dependent, differential development does occur. Often, specific deficits occur in a single dimension within a process, e.g., phonology, syntax, semantics, or pragmatics. The severity of specific deficits may vary, but experience at the Waisman Center has indicated that they are usually mild to moderate in degree. Severe deficits in one dimension are usually accompanied by deficits in other dimensions of the process, demonstrating their interdependence. In production, for example, phonological deficits resulting in a high proportion of unintelligible utterances will directly affect analysis of syntax and semantics. The interdependence of linguistic domains is at two levels: measurement and theoretical. At the measurement level, absence or deficits in one domain precludes analysis of other domains, as in the effect of phonological deficit on the analysis of inflectional development. At the theoretical level, achievements in syntax may be dependent upon achievements in semantic acquisition or phonology and syntax may employ similar processes in acquisition. Although experimental data have yet to demonstrate theoretical linkages between linguistic parameters within processes, clinically, care must be taken to distinguish between measurement limitations and limitations in the child's knowledge.

The final step in interpreting assessment data is to determine the developmental level of performance for each dimension evaluated using whatever criteria are available, e.g., test norms or developmental research data (see Chapters 2 and 4). Children's performance can then be summarized on a developmental format similar to those displayed in Figures 2 and 3. This developmental display provides the opportunity to compare dimensions assessed within processes as well as to contrast development across processes, in relation to both chronological age and cognitive development. In addition, the format provides the means for comparing performance across children or for the same child over time. The result is a summary of assessment data in an easy-to-read format.

[2]This section taken in part from Miller, 1978, pp. 310–313.

Children with developmental problems evidence differential development in cognitive behavior, language comprehension and production, and the use of language for communication. The description of the child's development for these processes provides the basis for interpreting the child's status for language development, as well as for developing and implementing appropriate treatment programs.

In Figures 2 and 3, representative children exemplify the potential relationships between chronological age and the developmental process dimensions of cognition, comprehension, production, and the use of language for communication. In Figures 2 and 3, individual children are represented by the letters A through H, where, reading across from left to right, the child's developmental status is displayed for each process. Any downward slope in the lines connecting the letters indicates a delay in that process in relation to chronological age.

Child A, for example, evidences cognitive development expected for his age, with comprehension and production also appropriate for his age. His use of language for communication is delayed, however. This developmental configuration is not uncommon in certain emotionally disturbed children and children who evidence communication problems only in certain situations.

Child B is delayed only in production of syntax. He uses what productive language he has for communication appropriately for his age.

Child C has appropriate cognitive development but shows delays in comprehension, production, and use at about the same level, as compared with child D whose delay in production is more pronounced than his delay in comprehension. Children with this pattern of development may evidence use of language compatible with either their comprehension or production development.

Children A through D (Figure 1) are all of normal intelligence but evidence different language problems. Their language performance can be interpreted as being delayed only on specific processes or on individual dimensions within these processes. Furthermore, some children are delayed on more than one process and some processes are more delayed than others (as in child D).

Children E through H (Figure 2) can be considered mentally retarded, given that their cognitive development is delayed, as measured psychometrically or within Piaget's developmental psychology. The development of language processes in these children is also differential as represented by children E, F, and G. The developmental patterns of each of these children are different, indicating that treatment considerations should be different for each child. Child H represents a paradox that is common among retarded children, particularly those living at home. The child's language comprehension, production, and use are consistent with his level of cognitive development. The question is, does this child have a language problem? This is and has been debatable, and no attempt is made to resolve the issue here. The illustration serves to point out that this and other similar questions have not been addressed in the experimental literature. This results in inconsistent decision-making about who should and should not receive treatment services or who could or could not benefit from a treatment program.

These summary displays describe only general development characteristics. The data required to generate the summaries must not be forgotten. These data comprise the detailed description of performance necessary to develop the content for teaching programs.

By determining the child's level of development on the processes necessary for acquisition and use, the degree to which other factors influence the child's performance can be determined. The environmental factors, for example, of a second language spoken in the home, limited language input from the parents, or institutional placement, may result in decreased performance on the processes evaluated in different ways. We have found that children with severe productive language deficits also have structural and functional problems with the speech production mechanism. Children with decreased hearing acuity will evidence delays in both comprehension and production of language. The relative influence of these factors must be determined on an individual basis. There is little direct evidence in the literature of the interactive nature of these factors with the processes affecting language acquisition.

INTERPRETATION RULES

The interpretation of multidimensional assessment data is an art as well as a science. It requires knowledge of developmental processes, relationships between dimensions, variables affecting performance, and factors affecting acquisition. In addition it requires judgment. The primary judgment required for interpretation is our confidence that the data reflect child performance. No amount of analysis will overcome the problem of lack of representativeness of the behaviors under study. Such judgments are basic to clinical practice. Before making pronouncements about children that may have far-reaching and sometimes irrevocable consequences, we must be

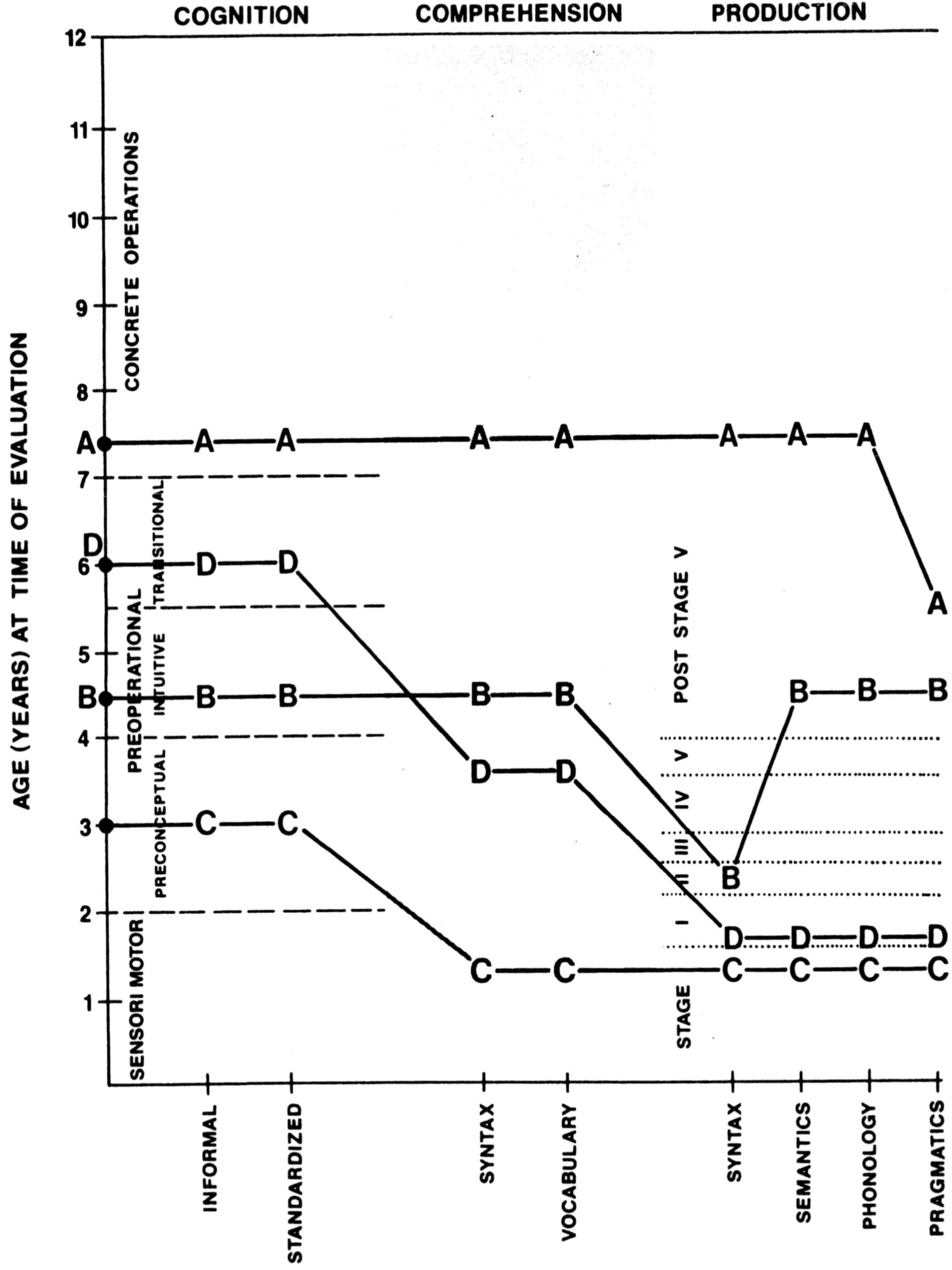

Figure 2. Some potential relationships between age and the developmental process dimensions: Children A–D.

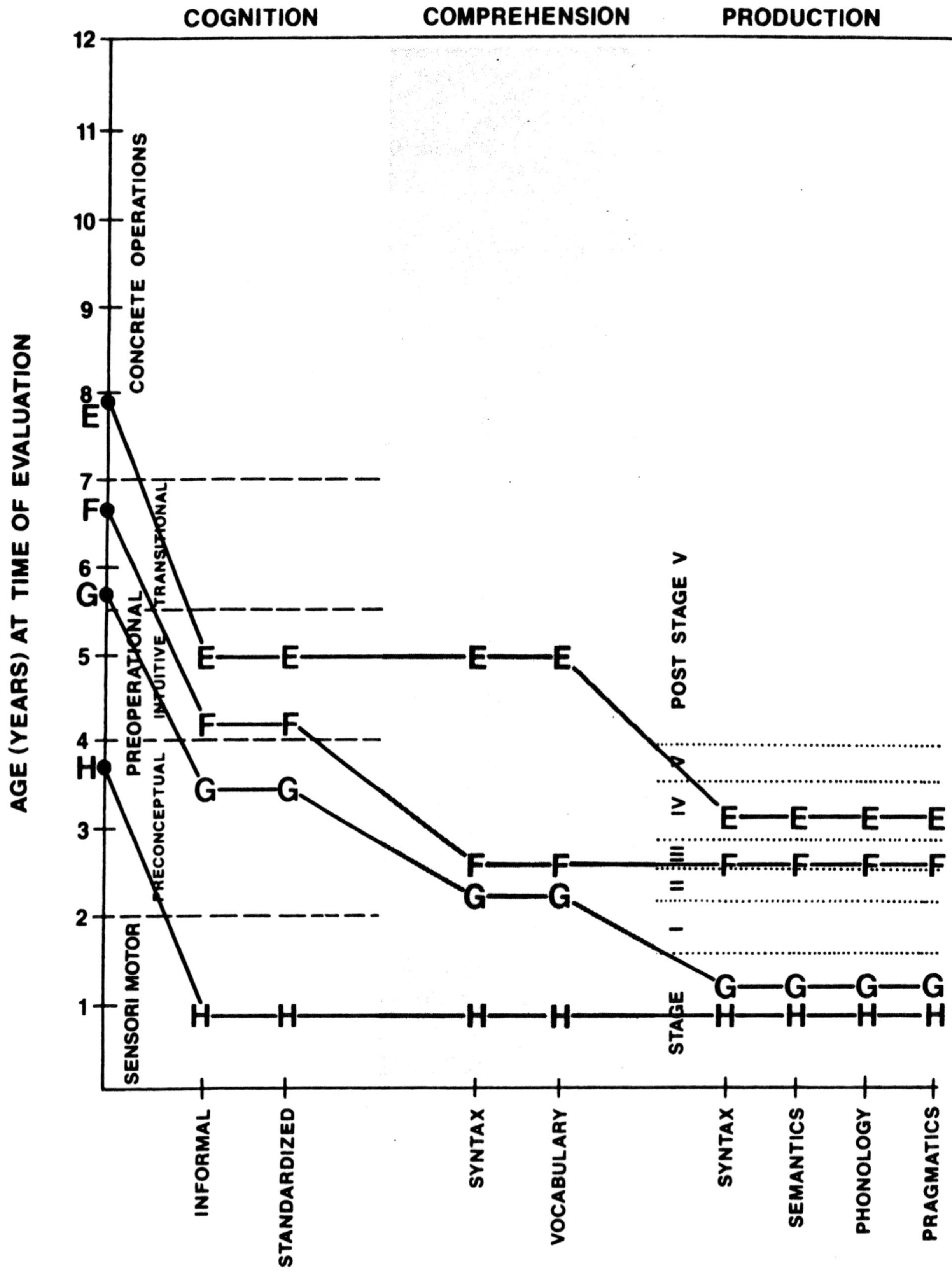

Figure 3. Some potential relationships between age and the developmental process dimensions: Children E–H.

certain that our data represent the facts about the child's communicative performance.

Two general rules regarding interpretation have served us well in minimizing precipitous decisions. The first rule is *never assume.* Never assume hearing is normal, vision is normal, speech motor control is normal, etc. Always gather performance data. The second rule is, once you have gathered some performance data, *assume it is wrong.* Do not trust the data from single recording sessions or single data points. Always look for confirming data by comparing the results of different procedures, for example, free-speech analysis versus elicited production of Wh-questions.

The application of these two rules sums to a skeptical view of data from single assessment sessions. While this may not be an appealing notion where time and effort are concerned, consider the impact of pragmatic parameters on performance. This alone should be sufficiently humbling to warrant extreme care in judging children to be normal or disordered speakers and listeners.

References

Akmajian, A., and Heny, F. 1975. An Introduction to the Principles of Transformational Syntax. The MIT Press, Cambridge, Mass.

Antinucci, F., and Parisi, D. 1976. Elements of Grammar. Academic Press, New York.

Austin, J. L. 1962. How to Do Things with Words. Harvard University Press, Cambridge, Mass.

Baldwin, A., and Baldwin, C. 1973. The study of mother-child interaction. Am. Sci. 61:714-721.

Bales, R. E. 1950. A set of categories for the analysis of small group interactions. Am. Sociol. Rev. 15:257-263.

Barlow, M., and Miner, L. 1969. Temporal reliability of Length-Complexity Index. J. Commun. Disord. 2:241-251.

Bates, E. 1976. Language and Context: The Acquisition of Pragmatics. Academic Press, New York.

Bates, E., Benigni, L., Bretherton, I., Camaioni, L., and Volterra, V. 1977. Cognition and Communication from 9-13 months: A correlational study. Report No. 12, Institute for the Study of Intellectual Behavior, University of Colorado, Boulder.

Bates, E., Benigni, L., Bretherton, I., Camaioni, L., and Volterra, V. 1979. The Emergence of Symbols: Cognition and Communication in Infancy. Academic Press, New York.

Bates, E., Camaioni, L., and Volterra, V. 1975. The acquisition of performatives prior to speech. Merrill-Palmer Q. 31:205-226.

Bates, E., and Johnston, J. 1978. The Development of Pragmatics. Short course presented at the Annual Convention of the American Speech and Hearing Association, Chicago, November 2-5, 1977.

Bellugi-Klima, U. 1968. Evaluating the child's language competence. Unpublished report No. ED-019-141. National Laboratory on Early Childhood Education, Washington, D.C.

Berry, P. (ed.), 1976. Language and Communication in the Mentally Handicapped. University Park Press, Baltimore.

Bloom, L. 1970. Language Development: Form and Function of Emerging Grammars. The MIT Press, Cambridge.

Bloom, L. 1973. One Word At A Time. Mouton, The Hague.

Bloom, L. 1974. Talking, understanding, and thinking. In R. L. Schiefelbusch and L. L. Lloyd (eds.), Language Perspectives—Acquisition, Retardation, and Intervention, pp. 285-311. PRO-ED, Inc., Austin.

Bloom, L., Hood, L., and Lightbown, P. 1974. Imitation in language development: If, when, and why. Cog. Psychol. 6:380-420.

Bloom, L., and Lahey, M. 1978. Language Development and Language Disorders. John Wiley and Sons, New York.

Bloom, L., Lahey, M., Hood, L., Lifter, K., and Fiess, K. Complex sentences: Acquisition of syntactic connectives and the semantic relations they encode. J. Child. Lang., In press.

Bloom, L., Lightbown, P., and Hood, L. 1973. Conventions for transcription of child language recordings. Unpublished paper, Teachers College, Columbia University, New York.

Bloom, L., Lightbown, P., and Hood, L. 1975. Structure and variation in child language. Monogr. Soc. Res. in Child Dev. 40:2.

Bloom, L., Rocissano, L., and Hood, L. 1976. Adult-child discourse: Developmental interaction between information processing and linguistic knowledge. Cog. Psychol. 8:521-552.

Bowerman, M. 1974. Discussion summary—Development of concepts underlying language. In R. L. Schiefelbusch and L. L. Lloyd (eds.), Language Perspectives—Acquisition, Retardation, and Intervention, pp. 191-209. PRO-ED, Inc., Austin.

Bowerman, M. 1978. Semantic and syntactic development: A review of what, when, and how in language acquisition. In R. Schiefelbusch (ed.), Bases of Language Intervention, pp. 97-189. University Park Press, Baltimore.

Bowerman, M. 1979. The acquisition of complex sentences. In P. Fletcher and M. Garman (eds.), Language Acquisition, pp. 285-305. Cambridge University Press, New York.

Braine, M. 1976. Children's first word combinations. Monograph Soc. Res. in Child Dev. 41:1.

Brown, H. D. 1971. Children's comprehension of relativized English sentences. Child Dev. 42:1923-1936.

Brown, R. 1973. A First Language. Harvard University Press, Cambridge, Mass.

Brown, R. 1970. The first sentences of child and chimpanzee. In R. Brown (ed.), Psycholinguistics. The Free Press, New York.

Brown, R., and Bellugi, U. 1964. Three processes in the child's acquisition of syntax. Harvard Educ. Rev. 34:2.

Bruner, J. 1975a. From communication to language: A psychological perspective. Cognition 3:255-287.

Bruner, J. 1975b. The ontogenesis of speech acts. J. Child Lang. 2:1-19.

Bruner, J. 1978. On prelinguistic prerequisites of speech. In R. N. Campbell and P. T. Smith (eds.), Recent Advances in the Psychology of Language, pp. 194-214, Vol. 4a. Plenum Press, New York.

Carrow, E. 1973. Test for auditory comprehension of language, English/Spanish versions. Urban Research Group, Austin, Tex.

Carrow, E. 1974. A test using elicited imitation in assessing grammatical structure in children. J. Speech and Hear. Disord. 39:437-444.

Cazden, C. 1968. The acquisition of noun and verb inflections. Child Devel. 39:433-438.

Chafe, W. 1970. Meaning and the Structure of Language. University of Chicago Press, Chicago.

Chapman, R. S. 1978, Personal Communication.

Chapman, R. S. Child language acquisition. In N. Lass, J. Northern, D. Yoder, and L. McReynolds (eds.), Speech, Hearing and Language. W. B. Saunders, Philadelphia. In press. a.

Chapman, R. S. Children's answers to Wh-questions. In J. Miller (ed.), Assessing Language Comprehension in Children: Experimental Procedures. University Park Press, Baltimore. In Preparation.

Chapman, R. S. Mother child interaction in the second year of life: Its Role in Language Development. In preparation a.

Chapman, R. S. Cognitive development and language comprehension in 10- to 21-month-olds. In R. Stark (ed.), Language Behavior in Infancy and Early Childhood. Elsevier North Holland Publishing Co., New York. In press. b.

Chapman, R. S., and Miller, J. F. 1975. Word order in early two and three word utterances: Does production precede comprehension? J. Speech Hear. Res. 18:355-371.

Chapman, R. S., and Miller, J. F. 1980. Analyzing language and communication in the child. In R. L. Schiefelbusch (ed.), Nonspeech Language and Communication, pp. 159-196. University Park Press, Baltimore.

Chapman, R. S., Paul, R., and Wanska, S. Syntactic structures in simple sentences. In preparation.

Clancy, P., Jacobsen, T., and Silva, M. 1976. The Acquisition of Conjunction: A Cross-Linguistic Study. Stanford University Committee on Linguistics, Papers Reports Child Lang. Dev. 12:71-80.

Clark, E. V. 1973. What's in a word? On the child's acquisition of semantics in his first language. In T. Moore (ed.), Cognitive Development and the Acquisition of Language, pp. 65-110. Academic Press, New York.

Coggins, T., and Carpenter, R. 1978. Categories for coding pre-speech intentional communication. Unpublished manuscript, University of Washington, Seattle.

Collis, G., and Schaffer, H. 1975. Synchronization of visual attention in mother-infant pairs. J. Child Psychol. Psychiatry 16(4):315-332.

Compton, A. 1970. Generative studies of children's phonological disorders. J. Speech Hear. Disord. 35:315-339.

Cromer, R. F. 1974. Receptive language in the mentally retarded: Processes and diagnostic distinction. In R. L. Schiefelbusch and L. L. Lloyd (eds.), Language Perspectives—Acquisition, Retardation, and Intervention, pp. 237-267. PRO-ED, Inc., Austin.

Cromer, R. F. 1976. The cognitive hypothesis of language acquisition for child language deficiency. In D. Morehead and A. Morehead (eds.), Normal and Deficient Child Language, pp. 283-333. University Park Press, Baltimore.

Crystal, D. 1979. Working with LARSP. Elsevier North Holland Publishing Co., New York.

Crystal, D., Fletcher, P., and Garman, M. 1976. The Grammatical Analysis of Language Disability: A Procedure for Assessment and Remediation. Elsevier-North Holland Publishing Co., New York.

Davison, A. 1974. Linguistic play and language acquisition. Stanford University Committee on Linguistics, Papers Reports Child Lang. Dev. 8:179-181.

DeArmengol, M., Goldstein, F., and Lombana, I. 1974. Comparison and imitation, comprehension and production of grammatical contrasts by children from high and low socio-economic classes. Rev. Lat. Am. Psicol. 6:239-254.

Dever, R. 1978. Teaching the American Language to Kids: Talk. Charles E. Merrill Publishing Co., Columbus.

Dever, R., and Bauman, P. 1974. Scale of children's clausal development. In T. M. Longhurst (ed.), Linguistic Analysis of Children's Speech, pp. 280-320. MCS Information Corporation, New York.

de Villiers, J., and de Villiers, P. 1973a. Development of the use of word order in comprehension. J. Psycholinguist. Res. 2(4):331-341.

de Villiers, J., and de Villiers, P. 1973b. A cross-sectional study of the acquisition of grammatical morphemes in child speech. J. Psycholinguist. Res. 2:267-268.

de Villiers, J., and de Villiers, P. 1978. Language Acquisition. Harvard University Press, Cambridge, Mass.

Dihoff, R. E., and Chapman, R. S. 1977. First words: Their origins in action. Stanford University Committee on Linguistics, Papers Reports Child Lang. Dev. 13:1-7.

Dore, J. 1974. A pragmatic description of early language development. J. Psycholinguist. Res. 4:343-350.

Dore, J. 1975. Holophrases, speech acts and language universals. J. Child Lang. 2:21-40.

Dore, J. 1976. Children's illocutionary acts. In R. Freedle (ed.), Discourse Relations: Comprehension and Production. Lawrence Erlbaum Associates, Hillsdale, N.J.

Dore, J. 1977. "Oh Them Sheriff": A pragmatic analysis of children's responses to questions. In S. Ervin-Tripp and C. Mitchell-Kernan (eds.), Child Discourse, pp. 139-164. Academic Press, New York.

Dore, J. 1978. Requestive systems in nursery school conversations: Analysis of talk in its social context. In R. Campbell and P. Smith (eds.), Recent Advances in the Psychology of Language: Language development and mother-child interaction. Plenum Press, New York.

Dunn, L. 1965. Peabody Picture Vocabulary Test. American Guidance Service, Inc., Circle Pines, Minn.

Engler, L., Hanna, E., and Longhurst, T. 1973. Linguistic analysis of speech samples: A practical guide for clinicians. J. Speech Hear. Disord. 38(2):192-204.

Ervin-Tripp, S. 1970. Discourse agreement: How children answer questions. In J. R. Hayes (ed.), Cognition and the Development of Language, pp. 79-108. John Wiley and Sons, New York.

Fillmore, C. 1968. Lexical entries for verbs. Foundations Lang. 4:373-393.

Fisher, M. 1934. Language patterns of preschool children. Child Dev. Monogr. No. 15.

Folger, J. P., and Chapman, R. S. 1978. A pragmatic analysis of spontaneous imitations. J. Child Lang. 5:25-38.

Folger, J. P., and Puck, S. 1976. Coding relational communication: A question approach. Paper presented at the International Communication Convention, Portland, Oregon.

Fraser, C., Bellugi, U., and Brown, R. 1963. Control of grammar in imitation and comprehension and production. J. Verb. Learn. Verb. Behav. 2:121-135.
Fromkin, V., and Rodman, R. 1974. An Introduction to Language. Holt, Rinehart and Winston, New York.
Garvey, C. 1975. Requests and responses in children's speech. J. Child Lang. 2:41-63.
Garvey, C. 1977. The contingent query. In M. Lewis and L. Rosenblum (eds.), Interaction, Conversation and the Development of Language, pp. 63-94. John Wiley and Sons, New York.
Goldin-Meadow, S., Seligman, M., and Gelman, R. 1976. Language in the two-year-old. Cognition 4:189-202.
Greenfield, P., and Smith, J. 1976. The Structure of Communication in Early Language Development. Academic Press, New York.
Grice, H. Logic and Conversation. William James Lecture, Harvard University, 1967. Portions of these lectures have been published in D. Davidson and G. Harmon, 1975. The Logic of Conversation. Dickensen Publishing Co., Encino, Calif.
Griffith, J., and Miner, L. 1969. LCI reliability and size of language sample. J. Commun. Disord. 2:264-267.
Halliday, M. A. K. 1975. Learning how to mean: Explorations in the development of language. Elsevier-North Holland Publishing Co., New York.
Hood, L., and Bloom, L. 1979. What, when and how about why: A longitudinal study of early expressions of causality. Monograph Soc. Res. in Child Dev., Serial 181.
Hood, L., Lahey, M., Lifter, K., and Bloom, L. 1978. Observational descriptive methodology in studying child language: Preliminary results on the development of complex sentences. In G. P. Sackett (ed.), Observing Behavior Vol. 1: Theory and Applications in Mental Retardation, pp. 239-263. University Park Press, Baltimore.
Hood, L., and Lightbown, P. 1978. What children do when asked to "Say what I say": Does elicited imitation measure linguistic knowledge? Allied Health Behav. Sci. 1(2):195-219.
Howe, C. 1976. The meaning of two-word utterances in the speech of young children. J. Child Lang. 3(1):29-47.
Huttenlocher, J. 1974. The origins of language comprehension. In R. L. Solso (ed.), Theories of Cognitive Psychology, pp. 331-368. Lawrence Erlbaum Associates, Hillsdale, N.J.
Ingram, D. 1971. Transitivity and Child Language. Language 47(4):888-910.
Ingram, D. 1972. The development of phrase structure rules. Lang. Learn. 22:65-77.
Ingram, D. 1974. Stages in the development of one word utterances. Paper presented at the Stanford Child Language Research Forum, April 1974, Stanford University, Stanford, Calif.
Ingram, D. 1975. If and when transformations are acquired by children. Monograph Series on Languages and Linguistics No. 27. Georgetown University, Washington, D.C.
Ingram, D. 1976. Phonological Disability in Children. Edward Arnold, London.
Ingram, D. 1979. Early patterns of grammatical development. Paper presented at Language Behavior in Infancy and Early Childhood Conference, Santa Barbara, Cal.
Ingram, D. Sensorimotor intelligence and language development. In A. Lock (ed.), Action, Gesture and Symbol: The Emergence of Language. Academic Press, New York. In press a.
Ingram, D. The transition from early symbols to syntax. In R. L. Schiefelbusch and D. Bricker (eds.), Early Language Intervention. University Park Press, Baltimore. In press b.
Ingram, D. 1981. Procedures For Phonological Analysis of Children's Language. University Park Press, Baltimore.
Inhelder, B. 1966. Cognitive development and its contributions to the diagnosis of some phenomena of mental deficiency. Merrill-Palmer Q. 12:299-319.
Inhelder, B. 1968. The Diagnosis of Reasoning in the Mentally Retarded. Chandler Publishing Company, New York.
Inhelder, B. 1976. Some pathologic phenomena analyzed in the perspective of developmental psychology. In B. Inhelder and H. Chapman (eds.), Piaget and His School. Springer-Verlag, New York.
James, S. 1978. Effect of listener age and situation on the politeness of children's directives. J. Psycholinguist. Res. 7:307-317.
Kahn, J. 1975. Relationship of Piaget's sensori-motor period to language acquisition of profoundly retarded children. Am. J. Mental Defic., 79, 640-643.
Keenan, E. O . 1977. Making it last: Repetition in children's discourse. In S. Ervin-Tripp and C. Mitchell-Kernan (eds.), Child Discourse, Academic Press, Inc., New York.
Klima, E., and Bellugi, U. 1966. Syntactic regularities in the speech of children. In J. Lyons and R. Wells (eds.), Psycholinguistic Papers. Edinburgh University Press, Edinburgh.
Kuczaj, S., and Maratsos, M. 1975. What children *can* say before they *will*. Merrill-Palmer Q. 21:89-111.
Labov, W. 1966. On the grammaticality of everyday speech. Paper presented at the Annual Meeting of the Linguistic Society of America. New York.
Labov, W. 1970. The logic of non-standard English. In F. Williams (ed.), Language and Poverty. Markham Publishing Company, Chicago.
Labov, W., and Fanshel, D. 1977. Therapeutic Discourse: Psychotherapy as Conversation. Academic Press, New York.
Lackner, J. R. 1968. A developmental study of language behavior in retarded children. Neuropsychologia 8:87-104.
Lakoff, R. 1973. The logic of politeness; or minding your p's and q's. In C. Corum, T. Smith-Clark, and A. Weiser (eds.), Papers from the Ninth Regional Meeting of the Chicago Linguistic Society. University of Chicago, Department of Linguistics, Chicago.
Lee, L. 1966. Developmental sentence types: A method for comparing normal and deviant syntactic development. J. Speech Hear. Disord. 31:311-330.
Lee, L. 1969, 1971. Northwestern Syntax Screening Test (NSST). Northwestern University Press, Evanston, Ill.
Lee, L. 1974. Developmental Sentence Analysis. Northwestern University Press, Evanston, Ill.
Leonard, L. B. 1978. On Redefining Language Disorders in Children. Paper presented at the Eighth Annual Mid-South Conference on Communicative Disorders, February, 1978, Memphis, Tennessee.
Lewis, D. 1978. The Secret Language of Your Child. St.

Martin's Press, New York.
Lewis, M. M. 1951. Infant Speech. Humanities Press, New York.
Lezine, I. 1973. The transition from sensorimotor to earliest symbolic function in early development. Early Dev. 51:221–228.
Loban, W. 1976. Language Development. National Council of Teachers of English. Champaign-Urbana, Ill.
Lovell, J., and Dixon, E. 1965. The growth of the control of grammar in imitation, comprehension and production. J. Child Psychol. Psychiatry 14:123–138.
McCarthy, D. 1930. The language development of the preschool child. Institute of Child Welfare Monograph Series No. 4. University of Minnesota Press, Minneapolis.
McCarthy, D. 1954. Language development in children. In L. Carmichael (ed.), Manual of Child Psychology. 2nd Ed. pp. 492–630. John Wiley and Sons, New York.
McCarthy, D. 1972. Manual for the McCarthy Scales of Children's Abilities. The Psychological Corporation, New York.
McManis, D. L. 1970. Conservation, seriation and transitivity performance by retarded and average individuals. Am. J. Ment. Defic. 74:784–791.
McReynolds, L. V., and Huston, K. A. 1971. A distinctive feature analysis of children's misarticulations. J. Speech Hear. Disord. 36:113–124.
Menn, L., and Haselkorn, S. 1977. Now you see it, now you don't: Tracing the development of communicative competence. Unpublished paper, Boston University.
Menyuk, P. 1963. A preliminary evaluation of grammatical capacity in children. J. Verb. Learn. Verb. Behav. 2:429–439.
Menyuk, P. 1969. Sentences Children Use. The MIT Press, Cambridge, Mass.
Menyuk, P. 1974. Early development of receptive language: From babbling to words. In R. L. Schiefelbusch and L. L. Lloyd (eds.), Language Perspectives—Acquisition, Retardation, and Intervention, pp. 213–235. PRO-ED, Inc., Austin.
Miller, J. F. 1973. Sentence imitation in preschool children. Lang. Speech 16:1–4.
Miller, J. F. 1976. Procedures for assessing children's language: A developmental process approach. Unpublished manuscript, University of Wisconsin-Madison.
Miller, J. F. 1978. Assessing children's language behavior: A developmental process approach. In R. L. Schiefelbusch (ed.), Bases of Language Intervention, pp. 269–318. University Park Press, Baltimore.
Miller, J. F., and Chapman, R. S. 1975. Length variables in sentence imitation. Lang. Speech 18:35–41.
Miller, J. F., and Chapman, R. S. 1979. The relation between age and mean length of utterance in morphemes. Unpublished manuscript, University of Wisconsin-Madison.
Miller, J. F., Chapman, R. S., and Bedrosian, J. L. 1977. Defining developmentally disabled subjects for research: The relationship between etiology, cognitive development and language and communicative performance. Paper presented at the Second Annual Boston University Conference on Language Development, October 1, Boston.
Miller, J. F., Chapman, R. S., and Bedrosian, J. L. 1978. Defining developmentally disabled subjects for research: The relationship between etiology, cognitive development and communicative performance. New Zealand Speech Therapist's J. 33:2.
Miller, J. F., Chapman, R. S., Branston, M., and Reichle, J. 1980. Comprehension development in sensorimotor stages 5 and 6. J. Speech Hear. Res. 23:2.
Miller, J. F., and Yoder, D. 1972. The Miller-Yoder Test of Grammatical Comprehension, experimental edition (M-Y Test). University of Wisconsin-Madison (Bookstore).
Miller, J. F., and Yoder, D. 1973. Assessing the comprehension of grammatical form in mentally retarded children. Paper presented at the International Association for the Scientific Study of Mental Deficiency, The Hague, Netherlands, September, 1973.
Miller, J. F., and Yoder, D. The Miller-Yoder Test of Grammatical Comprehension. In J. F. Miller (ed.), Assessing Language Comprehension in Children: Experimental Procedures. University Park Press, Baltimore. In preparation.
Miner, L. 1969. Scoring procedures for the length complexity index: A preliminary report. J. Commun. Disord. 2:224–250.
Minifie, F., Darley, F., and Sherman, D. 1963. Temporal reliability of seven language measures. J. Speech Hear. Res. 6:139–148.
Moerk, E. L. 1975. Verbal interactions between children and their mothers during the preschool years. Dev. Psychol. 11:788–795.
Morehead, D. M., and Ingram, D. 1973. The development of base syntax in normal and linguistically deviant children. J. Speech Hear. Res. 16:330–352.
Morehead, D., and Morehead, A. 1974. From signal to sign: A Piagetian view of thought and language during the first two years. In R. L. Schiefelbusch and L. L. Lloyd (eds.), Language Perspectives—Acquisition, Retardation and Intervention, pp. 153–190. PRO-ED, Inc., Austin.
Muma, J. 1973. Language assessment: The co-occurring and restricted structure procedure. Acta Symbolica 4:12–29.
Nelson, K. 1973. Structure and strategy in learning to talk. Monogr. Soc. Res. Child Dev. 38, No. 149.
Ninio, A., and Bruner, J. 1978. The achievement and antecedents of labeling. J. Child Lang. 5(1):1–16.
Owings, N. O. 1972. Internal reliability and item analysis of the Miller-Yoder Test of Grammatical Comprehension. Unpublished master's thesis, University of Wisconsin-Madison.
Parten, M. 1933. Social play among preschool children. J. Abnorm. Soc. Psychol. 28:136–147.
Pea, R. 1978. Early Negation: The development from relating inner states to comments on the external world. Paper presented at the 3rd Annual Boston University Conference on Language Development, September, 1978, Boston.
Piaget, J. 1926. The Language and Thought of the Child. Harcourt, Brace, New York.
Piaget, J., and Inhelder, B. 1969. The Psychology of the Child. Basic Books, New York.
Pollack, E., and Rees, N. 1972. Disorders of articulation: Some clinical applications of distinctive feature theory. J. Speech Hear. Disord. 37:451–461.
Ratner, N., and Bruner, J. 1978. Games, social exchange and the acquisition of language. J. Child Lang. 5(3):391–402.

Retherford, K., Schwartz, B., and Chapman, R. Semantic roles in mother and child speech: Who tunes into whom? J. Child Lang. In press.
Ricks, D. M. 1975. Vocal communication in pre-verbal normal and autistic children. In N. O'Connor (ed.), Language, Cognitive Deficits, and Retardation. Butterworths, London.
Rogers, S. J. 1977. Characteristics of the cognitive development of profoundly retarded children. Child Dev. 48:837-843.
Rohiver, W. 1970. Images and pictures in children's learning: Research results and educational implications. Psychol. Bull. 73:393-403.
Rondal, J. 1978. Maternal speech to normal and Down's syndrome children matched for mean utterance length. In C. E. Meyers (ed.), Quality of Life in Severely and Profoundly Mentally Retarded People: Research Foundations for Improvement. American Association on Mental Deficiency, Washington, D.C.
Sachs, J., and Devin, J. 1973. Young children's knowledge of age-appropriate speech styles. Paper presented at the Annual Meeting of the Linguistic Society of America, December, 1973.
Sachs, J., and Truswell, L. 1976. Comprehension of two word instructions by children in the one-word stage. Paper presented at the 8th annual Stanford Child Language Research Forum, April 1976, Stanford University, Stanford, Calif.
Scaife, M., and Bruner, J. 1975. The capacity for joint visual attention in the infant. Nature 253(5489):265-266.
Schane, S. 1973. Generative Phonology. Prentice-Hall, Englewood Cliffs, N.J.
Scherer, N., and Coggins, T. Contingent responses to adult-initiated requests in the dialogues of stage I children. University of Washington, Seattle. In preparation.
Schlesinger, I. M. 1971. Learning grammar: From pivot to realization rule. In R. Huxley and E. Ingram (eds.), Language Acquisition: Models and Methods. Academic Press, New York.
Searle, J. 1969. Speech Acts. Cambridge University Press, Cambridge, Mass.
Searle, J. 1976. A classification of illocutionary acts. Lang. Soc. 5:1-23.
Seitz, S., and Stewart, C. 1975. Expanding on expansions and related aspects of mother-child communication. Dev. Psychol. 11:760-763.
Shriberg, L., and Kwiatkowski, J. 1980. Natural Process Analysis: A Procedure for Phonological Analysis of Continuous Speech Samples. John Wiley and Sons, New York.
Shriner, T. 1967. A comparison of selected measures with psychological scale values of language development. J. Speech Hear. Res. 10:828-835.
Shriner, T. 1969. A review of mean length of response as a measure of expressive language development in children. J. Speech Hear. Disord. 34:61-68.
Siegel, G. M., and Broen, P. A. 1976. Language assessment. In L. L. Lloyd (ed.), Communication Assessment and Intervention Strategies, pp. 73-122. University Park Press, Baltimore.
Singer, J. L. 1973. The Child's World of Make-Believe. Academic Press, New York.
Slobin, D. (ed.) 1967. A Field Manual for Cross-Cultural Study of the Acquisition of Communicative Competence. University of California Press, Berkeley.
Slobin, D. I. 1973. Cognitive prerequisites for the development of grammar. In C. A. Ferguson and D. I. Slobin (eds.), Studies of Child Language Development. Holt, Rinehart and Winston, New York.
Slobin, D., and Welsh, C. A. 1973. Elicited imitations as a research tool in developmental psycholinguistics. In C. A. Ferguson and D. I. Slobin (eds.), Studies in Child Language Acquisition. Holt, Rinehart, and Winston, New York.
Slosson, R. 1974. Slosson Intelligence Test (SIT) for children and adults. Western Psychological Services, Los Angeles.
Smith, C. 1970. An experimental approach to children's linguistic competence. In J. Hayes (ed.), Cognition and the Development of Language. John Wiley and Sons, New York.
Snyder, L. 1975. Pragmatics in language-disabled children: Their prelinguistic and early verbal performantives and presuppositions. Unpublished doctoral dissertation, University of Colorado.
Templin, M. C. 1957. Certain language skills in children: Their development and interrelationships. Child Welfare Monog. No. 26. University of Minnesota Press, Minneapolis.
Tough, J. 1977. The Development of Meaning. Halsted Press, New York.
Tyack, D., and Gottsleben, R. 1974. Language Sampling, Analysis and Training. Consulting Psychologists Press, Palo Alto, Calif.
Tyack, D., and Ingram, D. 1977. Children's production and comprehension of questions. J. Child Lang. 4(2):211-224.
Uzgiris, I., and Hunt, J. McV. 1975. Assessment in Infancy. University of Illinois Press, Urbana.
Vygotsky, L. S. 1962. Thought and Language. The MIT Press, Cambridge.
Wells, G. 1975. Learning to code experience through language. J. Child Lang. 1:243-269.
Wohlhueter, M. J., and Sindberg, R. M. 1975. Longitudinal development of object permanence in mentally retarded children: An exploratory study. Am. J. Ment. Defic. 79(5):513-518.
Wolfram, W., and Fasold, R. 1974. The Study of Social Dialects in American English. Prentice-Hall, Englewood Cliffs, N.J.
Woodward, M. 1959. The behavior of idiots interpreted by Piaget's theory of sensorimotor development. Br. J. Educ. Psychol. 29:60-71.
Woodward, M. 1961. Concepts of number of the mentally subnormal studied by Piaget's method. J. Child Psychol. Psychiatry 2:249-259.
Yoder, D. E., and Miller, J. F. 1972. What we may know and what we can do: Input toward a system. In J. McLean, D. Yoder and R. Schiefelbusch (eds.), Language Intervention with the Retarded, pp. 89-110. University Park Press, Baltimore.
Zigler, E. 1969. Developmental versus difference theories of mental retardation and the problem of motivation. Am. J. Ment. Defic. 73:536-556.

Index of Procedures

Subject Index